# Fatty Liver Cookbook

## 87 Effective Fatty Liver Diet Recipes Plus Guide To Reverse And Prevent Fatty Liver

SHARON WALTERS

# DEDICATION

For Uncle Miller,

Love you now and always!

*Suzanne*

# TABLE OF CONTENTS

# INTRODUCTION

## The Liver

The liver is a glandular organ of the body, located at the upper right-hand position below the diaphragm; it is protected by the ribs. The upper part of the liver is located close to the nipples and the lower part close to the stomach. It is one of the most versatile organs with a range of functions, although still being explored, there are about 400 functions associated with the liver, and the major functions include:

**The production of Bile**: Bile is a green substance which helps the small intestine in the breakdown and digestion of fats, vitamins and cholesterol.

**Albumin Production**: This is one of the most common protein contained in the blood serum. It transports steroid hormones and fatty acid to help regulate blood pressure and prevent the leaking of blood vessels

**Fat Metabolizing**: Through the creation of Bile, fats are broken down and become easier to digest.

**Carbohydrates Metabolizing**: When carbohydrates are broken down into glucose, they are stored in the liver as glycogen and transported throughout the body whenever a quick burst of energy is needed. They also help maintain normal glucose levels in the bloodstream as well as perform:

- Immunological function
- Protein metabolizing
- Immunological function
- Vitamin and mineral storage:

**Regulating Blood Clotting**: Bile is necessary for vitamin K, (a vitamin necessary for producing 4 of the 13 essential proteins that thicken the blood and prevent it from bleeding excessively

**Clearance Of Bilirubin:** The buildup of bilirubin in the blood turns the eyes and skin yellow

**Regenerative Function;** The regenerative function of the liver is one of the most remarkable qualities of the liver. The liver is the only visceral organ that is able to replace lost tissue and regenerate. 25% of the liver tissue is sufficient to renew growth and regenerate to the previous size.

### Duration Of Liver Regeneration
Although experts are yet to identify what makes a liver grow despite losing a large amount of tissue, it has been observed that the liver grows at a fast rate from as little as 3 weeks to 2 months before regenerating to its full size. However, liver regeneration is possible when a healthy diet that aids detoxification and boosts its capacity to heal itself is followed.

## Fatty Liver
Fatty liver or hepatic steatosis, is a condition where there is an excess of fat in the liver cells. The liver naturally contains small amounts of fat, however when there is a buildup of fatty tissues above 5% of the livers total weight, this would be considered a fatty liver.

In simple and mild forms, fatty liver is harmless and has no symptoms. It does not lead to liver damage and medical complications, but with a steady accumulation of fat, damage to the liver becomes severe and the liver becomes vulnerable to medical complications like inflammation which leads to hardening and scarring of the liver, a condition called *cirrhosis*.

Symptoms of an inflamed liver include:

- Weight loss
- Abdominal pain
- Confusion
- Fatigue

- Loss of appetite

When Cirrhosis develops and the damage becomes severe, it may lead to liver damage and subsequently, liver failure. Symptoms of Cirrhosis include:

Jaundice (yellowing of the skin), an effect of the accumulation of bilirubin in the blood

- Weakness
- Itching
- Fatigue
- Weight loss
- Easy bruising

With Cirrhosis present, the liver fails to carry out its function and the chemicals, waste product and toxins present in the body build up in the body. Without immediate attention, this may lead to multiple organ failure and eventually death.

## Types Of Fatty Liver

There are two main types of fatty liver

- Alcohol Related Fatty liver disease
- Non alcoholic Fatty liver disease.

# Non-alcoholic fatty liver disease.(NAFLD)

**Non-alcoholic fatty liver disease** is a term used to categorize the wide range of fatty liver conditions affecting individuals who take little or no amounts of alcohol, it occurs when there is a buildup of fat in the liver cells and the liver has difficult

**Nonalcoholic steatohepatitis** (NASH) is a form of Non-alcoholic fatty liver disease marked by a progression of fat above 5% in the liver tissue and subsequent inflammation. If left untreated, NASH can progress to permanent scarring of the liver, liver cancer, cirrhosis and eventual liver failure.

NASH occurs in every age group, however according to the **American liver foundation**, most cases of NASH are detected in people between the ages of 40 to 60. This is linked to a metabolic syndrome where all or more of the following conditions are present in the individuals of those age groups;

- Increase in abdominal fat

- Obesity

- Inability to use insulin/ Insulin resistance of the body

- High blood pressure

- Diabetes

- High level of blood fats (hyperlipidaemia)

# Alcohol Related Fatty Liver Disease

As the name implies, this form of fatty liver disease is caused by alcohol abuse. Alcohol abuse implies anyone drinking more than 15 alcoholic beverages per week consistently. Constant alcohol abuse leads to liver damage as the liver becomes weak and it becomes more and more difficult to break down toxins and fats. This can result in inflammation (alcoholic hepatitis), and scarring of the liver (cirrhosis).

Alcohol Related Fatty liver disease is made worse by poor diet, lack of exercise, the presence of preexisting medical conditions such as hepatitis C etc. However, alcohol related fatty liver is easy to reverse. It involves a series of changes which includes;

- Stop drinking
- Frequent exercise
- Weight loss
- Controlling blood sugar
- Managing amount of cholesterol in food and beverages

# Reversing Fatty liver

**What to Eat To Promote Fatty Liver Reversal**

1. Coffee: The presence of caffeine in coffee helps reduce the amount of abnormal liver enzymes present. Research has shown that regular coffee drinkers experience less liver damage than those who do not drink caffeinated beverages.

2. Low-Fat Dairy: Whey protein is known to help to protect the liver and huge amounts of this can be found in low-fat dairy such as Greek yoghurt

3. Fresh Fruits and Vegetables; Fruits and vegetables have been shown to aid in preventing the buildup of fats in the liver, they also provide fats essential vitamin and minerals that are beneficial to the general wellbeing of

the body. Fruits like papaya, broccoli, cherries, blueberries, tomatoes and other fruits are excellent sources.

4. Garlic: Garlic especially in powder supplements assist in reducing bodyweight

5. Fish and Animal Protein: Fatty fish such as Trout, sardines and salmon are rich in omega-3 fatty acids which help in reducing inflammation and fat levels in the liver. Poultry, Eggs, Turkey are examples of rich sources of animal protein.

6. Plant Protein: Protein assists in balancing the insulin levels and can help reduce the buildup of fatty tissues in the liver; soy protein is a rich source of plant protein which can be found in tofu. Tofu contains high amounts of protein and low fat.

7. Healthy Oils: Olive oils, Avocado oils, Coconut oils are all examples oils rich in omega-3 fatty acids, they are healthier for cooking and aid in reducing enzyme levels present in the liver, inflammation and maintaining a good body weight.

8. Whole Grains

9. Tea: Research shows that teas, especially green tea has numerous benefits, among which include lowering cholesterol, helpful interference with fat absorption and aiding with sleep.

10. Nuts and Seeds: These contain a lot of a lot of antioxidants, vitamins and omega-3 fatty acids which help protect the liver and improve its function. Examples are sunflower seeds, walnuts, Chia seeds, Flax seeds and more.

## Foods to Avoid or Limit

1. Alcohol: it impairs the livers ability and in excess, leads to fatty liver disease

2. Fried foods: they have high calorie content and promote unhealthy weight gain.

3. Added sugar: Asides lacking nutritional value, added sugar found in beverages and sugary drinks are the major contributors to the increase in fatty liver today. Sugar activates lipogenesis- the formation of fatty acids in the body, limit the amount of sugar in foods by checking labels and nutritional value of food and drinks, substitute sugary fruit and drinks for natural fruits which contain a healthy combination of juice and fiber.

4. High Glycemic Carbohydrates: This means carbohydrates that break down quickly into sugar; they are usually low in fiber and lead to the buildup of fat and development of insulin resistance in the liver. A healthy tip is to cut down on the consumption of processed foods.

5. Salt And Red Meat: The recommended salt intake is 1,500 milligrams per day. When possible, substitute salt for spices and herbs. Furthermore, beef and other forms of red meat have a high level of unsaturated fat which is not healthy for the liver.


Healthy Lifestyle Changes To Incorporate

1. Exercise: exercise is an effective way to deal with a fatty liver, regular exercise helps in weight loss, improves insulin resistance and helps burn triglycerides, all of which help to improve the general liver condition.

2. Avoid alcohol: this also applies to non-alcoholic fatty liver disease

3. Reduce or Stop Smoking: Smoking apart from the health implications to the lungs and heart also worsens fatty liver disease.

4. Lower cholesterol

5. Sufficient Sleep.

# BREAKFAST

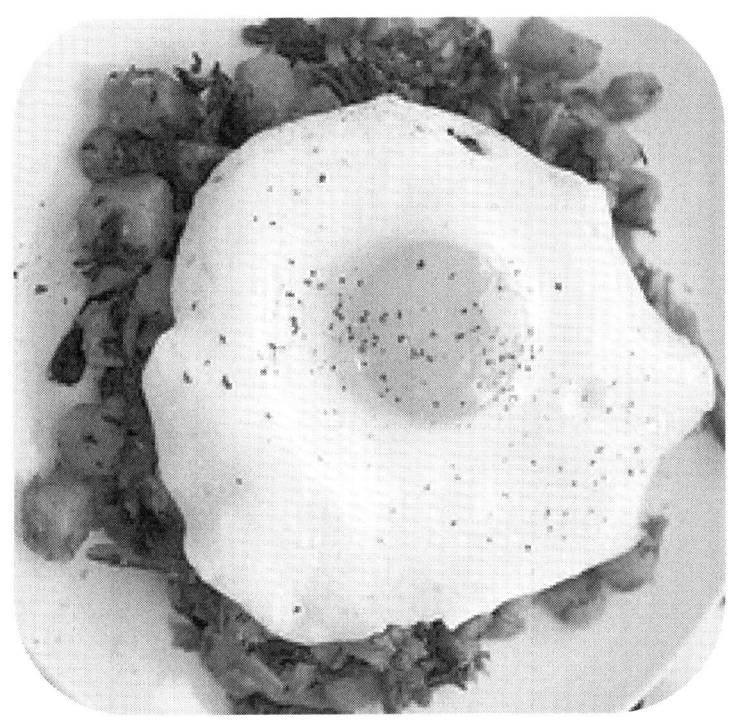

*Mexican Sweet Potato Hash with Black Beans and Spinach*

# Chia Greek Yogurt Pudding

Yields: 4 servings

Preparation time: 45 minutes

**Ingredients:**

1 cup unsweetened soy milk

1 cup Greek yogurt

2 tbsp of ground flax seeds

1 tbsp of honey

1 tsp of ground cinnamon

1 tsp of vanilla extract

1/3 cup chia seeds

**Instructions:**

1. Add soy milk and Greek yoghurt into a bowl, whisk until well combined, afterwards add honey, cinnamon, flax seeds and vanilla extract into the mixture, transfer mixture to a sealable jar and refrigerate for 15 minutes.

2. After 15 minutes, remove refrigerated jar and vigorously stir chia seeds to distribute them evenly, cover and refrigerate for 30 minutes until set. Serve and enjoy!

## Mexican Sweet Potato Hash with Black Beans and Spinach

Yields: 4 servings

Preparation time: 10 minutes

Cooking time: 25 minutes

**Ingredients:**

2 peeled medium sized sweet potatoes, cut into ½ inch cubes

1 large shallot, sliced thinly

1 15-ounce can black beans, drained and rinsed

1 tsp of sea salt

5 oz of baby spinach

2 tbsp of olive oil

½ tsp of ground cumin

½ tsp of chili powder

1 tbsp of lime juice

Eggs, optional

**Instructions:**

1. Heat olive oil in a large sized skillet over medium heat, afterwards add the potatoes and cook for about 15 minutes until tender and brown, stir regularly.

2. Next, add in black beans, cumin, chili powder and salt. Cook until the shallot turns soft, this takes about 3 minutes, stir in spinach and cook until it turns wilted.

3. Reduce heat to low, add a drizzle of lime juice and simmer for 5 minutes. Serve warm layered with fried egg, enjoy!

# Fluffiest Blueberry Pancakes

Yields: 6-8 large thick pancakes

Preparation time: 10 minutes

Cooking time: 10 minutes

**Ingredients:**

3/4 cup milk

2 tbsp of white vinegar

1 cup flour

2 tbsp of sugar

1 tsp of baking powder

1/2 tsp of salt

1/2 tsp of baking soda

1 egg

2 tbsp of melted butter + 1 tsp for the skillet

1 cup of blueberries

**Instructions:**

1. In a large bowl, add milk and vinegar, stir until smooth, set aside to sit for 1 minute.

2. Evenly spread the teaspoon of butter into the skillet. Add flour, salt, sugar, baking powder and baking soda to the milk and vinegar mixture and stir to combine well.

3. Next, add the egg, 2 tablespoons of butter and milk, stir..

4. Place skillet over heat set to medium, Stir in 1/3 of the batter, add a few pieces of blueberries and cook until the edges turn firm and you see bubbles, flip and cook until crisp. Enjoy!

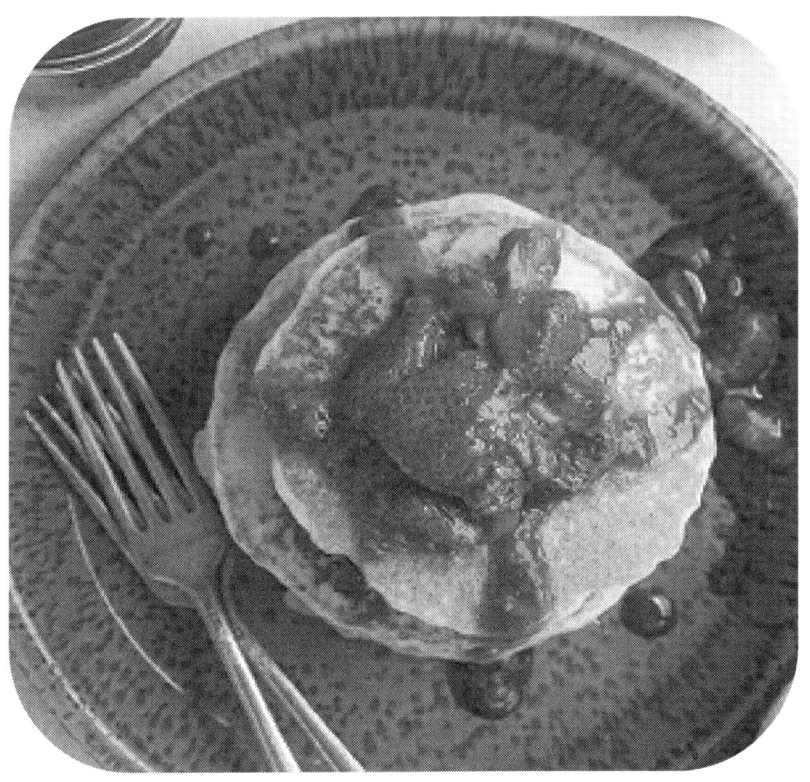

*Almond Milk Pancakes*

# Almond Milk Pancakes

Yields: 14 small pancakes

Preparation time: 5 minutes

Cooking time: 10 minutes

**Ingredients:**

1 ½ cups of all-purpose flour,

2 tbsp of sugar

1 tsp of baking powder

1 ¼ cups almond milk

2 tbsp of oil

1 egg

A pinch of salt

1 tbsp of melted butter, for the skillet

Strawberries (topping)

**Instructions:**

1. In a large bowl, add in the flour, sugar, baking powder and salt, stir until smooth

2. Add the egg, milk, oil and stir. Afterwards, place skillet over low-medium heat, add butter and heat.

3. Next, stir in batter. And cook until the edges turn firm and you see bubbles, flip and heat until evenly cooked.

4. Serve pancakes on a plate and layer with a sprinkle of powdered sugar and strawberry toppings. Enjoy!

# Almond Milk Oatmeal

Yields: 4 servings

Preparation time: 5 minutes

Cooking time: 5 minutes

**Ingredients:**

2 cups almond milk, unsweetened

¼   teaspoon of salt

1 cup of dry rolled oats

**Instructions:**

1. Pour the salt and almond milk into a medium sized saucepan placed over low-medium heat and boil, stir regularly.

2.  Add in the oats and cook for about 3 to 5 minutes, enjoy!


# Mixed Berry Vanilla Baked Oatmeal

Yields: 6 servings

Preparation time: 20 minutes

Cooking time: 35 minutes

Ingredients:

3 cups old fashioned rolled oats

1 1/2 tsp of baking powder

1/2 tsp of salt

2 eggs, beaten

2 1/2 cups of coconut milk

1/2 cup maple syrup

2 tsp of pure vanilla extract

3 tbsp of coconut oil, melted + 1 tsp to grease baking dish

3 cups fresh strawberries and raspberries, chopped

**Instructions:**

1. Lightly grease a 3 quart baking dish with the teaspoon of oil , set oven temperature to 350°F.

2. Next, add the baking powder, oats and salts into a bowl and stir to combine well, set aside. In another bowl, stir in the maple syrup, eggs, vanilla extract and coconut oil, set aside.

3. Transfer half of the oats mixture into the oiled baking dish, layer mixture with half of the berries and top with the other half of the oat mixture.

4. Pour the maple syrup mixture over the oats and top with a sprinkle of the remaining berries. Bake uncovered for about 30 minutes or more, until oats are tender and set, Enjoy!

# Quinoa Porridge

Yields: 2 servings

Preparation time: 10 minutes

Cooking time: 20 minutes

**Ingredients:**

1/2 cup quinoa

1/4 tsp of ground cinnamon

1 tsp of vanilla extract

1/2 cups of almond milk

1/2 cup water

A pinch of salt

2 tbsp of brown sugar

**Instructions:**

1. Place the quinoa into a saucepan over low-medium heat, season with ground cinnamon and cook for about 5 minutes until toasted, stir frequently.

2. Stir in the last 5 ingredients and cook for about 25 minutes until the porridge turns thick, add water to reach desired consistency if preferred. Stir regularly.

# Gluten Free Sweet Potato Waffles

Yields: 8 Servings

Preparation time: 10 minutes

Cooking time: 10 minutes

**Ingredients:**

2 cups Sweet potato puree

2 Eggs, beaten

1 cup of milk

2 cups gluten-free oats

2 teaspoon of Baking powder

1 tsp Vanilla extract

1 teaspoon of Baking soda

1 teaspoon of Cinnamon

1/2 teaspoon of ground Nutmeg

**Instructions**

1. Add all ingredients to a blender and blend until completely smooth.

2. Lightly grease and preheat the waffle iron , spoon waffle mixture into the iron mold of the  waffle iron and cook for about 5 minutes until it becomes golden on both ends

3. Transfer to a plate and enjoy with maple syrup if desired

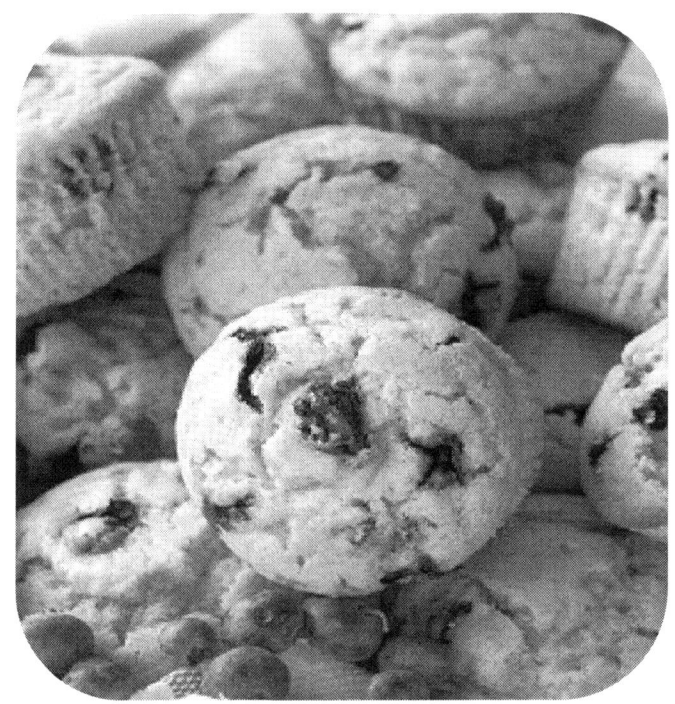
*Blueberry Oatmeal Muffins*

# Blueberry Oatmeal Muffins

Yields: 16 muffins

Preparation time: 15 minutes

Cooking time: 25 minutes

**Ingredients:**

2 large eggs

1 2/3 cups of quick-cooking oats

3/4 tsp of salt

1/2 cup of whole-wheat flour

3/4 cup of brown sugar

2 tsp of ground cinnamon

1 tsp of baking powder

1 tsp of baking soda

2/3 cup of almond flour

1 1/2 cups of low-fat buttermilk

1/4 cup of canola oil

2 tsp of lemon rind, grated

2 cups blueberries, frozen

2 tbsp of all-purpose flour Cooking spray

2 tbsp of granulated sugar

**Instructions:**

1. Preheat the oven to 400°F, pour oats into a food processor and blend until oats turn coarse.

2. Combine the wheat and almond flour in a large bowl, add the oats, baking powder, soda, lemon rind and cinnamon

3. Next, combine buttermilk and the remaining ingredients into a bowl, stir well and then transfer into the flour mixture, stir once more until moist.

4. Add the berries and stir to distribute evenly. Spoon batter into cups and coat the cups with all purpose flour cooking spray.

5. Drizzle sugar over the distributed batter, transfer to preheated oven and bake for about 20 minutes, check for doneness by touching muffins lightly in the middle, they should spring up when done. Enjoy!

# Turkey Lettuce Wraps

Yields: 6 servings.

Preparation time: 10 minutes

Cooking time: 10 minutes

**Ingredients:**

1¼ pound lean ground turkey, fat-free

1 tablespoon of olive oil

1 clove of minced garlic

1/8 teaspoon ground ginger

4 green onions, sliced thinly

1 (8 oz) can water chestnuts, chopped coarsely and drained

3 tablespoon of hoisin sauce

2 tablespoon of lower-sodium soy sauce

1 tablespoon of rice vinegar

2 teaspoon of red chili paste, roasted

Pinch of salt

12 Boston lettuce leaves

**Instructions:**

1. Spread olive oil a large sized skillet set on low-medium heat, add the garlic, ginger and turkey and cook until the turkey turns brown, this takes about 5 minutes.

2. Transfer turkey mixture into a large bowl, add onions and chestnuts and stir to combine well.

3. Using a separate small bowl, mix and stir rice vinegar, hoisin, soy sauce and chili paste, transfer to the owl containing the lettuce mixture and toss to combine.

4. Divide turkey mixture and share equally to each lettuce leaf, serve and enjoy!

## Coconut Chia Porridge

Yields: 4 Servings

Preparation time: 5 minutes

Cooking time: 5 minutes

**Ingredients:**

4 cup of almond milk

4 tablespoon of ground flax seed

4 tablespoon of chia seeds

4 tablespoon of hemp seeds

1 cup shredded coconut, unsweetened

A pinch of sea salt

4 vanilla bean

Honey and pistachios dried figs, to garnish

**Instructions:**

1. Slice vanilla bean and scrape seeds into the almond milk ,pour the almond milk into a small saucepan with heat set to medium and boil.

2. After milk boils, reduce heat to low and add the shredded coconut, flax, hemp and chia seeds, stir. Taste and add salt as desired, cook until the porridge thickens.

3. Transfer to plates and serve garnished with figs and a light drizzle of honey. Enjoy!

# Coconut Granola

Yields: 5 granola cups

Preparation time: 10 minutes

Cooking time: 30 minutes

**Ingredients:**

2 cups old-fashioned oats

1/3 cup pepitas

3/4 cup sweetened coconut, shredded

1/2 cup almonds, chopped

1 tsp of cinnamon

1/4 tsp of salt

4 tbsp of coconut oil, melted

1/2 cup maple syrup

1 tsp of vanilla extract

1/4 tsp of coconut extract

**Instructions:**

1. Preheat the oven to 300 F. Line a large baking sheet with parchment paper. Set aside.

2. Add first 6 ingredients into a large bowl and stir to combine, In a smaller bowl, whisk the last 4 ingredients, Transfer the contents of the small bowl into the larger bowl and stir until well coated.

3. Spread granola mixture in an even and consistent layer onto the baking sheet and bake until it turns golden brown, this would take about 30 minutes, stir at 10 minute intervals. Remove from the oven, cool and serve. Enjoy!

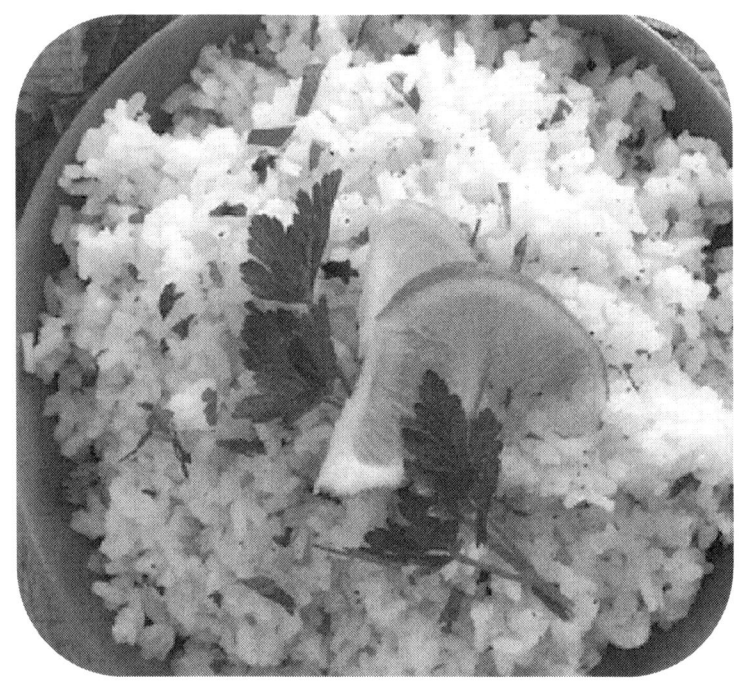

Cilantro Garlic Lime Rice

# Cilantro Garlic Lime Rice

Yields: 4 servings

Preparation time: 5 minutes

Cooking time: 20 minutes

**Ingredients:**

2 cups of Minute Rice

1 14 oz can of chicken broth

1/4 cup of limeade

1 1/2 tbsp of garlic, minced

1 1/2 tbsp of dried cilantro

**Instructions:**

1. Add broth and limeade into a medium-sized saucepan set over medium-high heat and bring to a boil.

2. Stir in the garlic, cilantro and rice and cook for about 10 minutes until done

3. Remove saucepan from heat, stand covered for about 5 minutes. Serve, enjoy!

# Apple Walnut Rice Stuffing

Yields: 4 servings

Preparation time: 10 minutes

Cooking time: 40 minutes

Ingredients:

1 cup of wild rice

2 tbsp of olive oil

1 small white onion, chopped finely

2 tbsp of olive oil

2 tbsp of port wine

1 tsp  parsley, dried

1/4 cup walnuts, chopped

2 McIntosh apples, cored and chopped

1 celery heart, minced

Salt

**Instructions:**

1. Pour 2 cups of water into a medium sized saucepan over medium heat, add oil, rice  and pinch of salt. Stir and cook for about 15-20 minutes.

2.  While rice boils, heat the olive oil in a skillet and sauté onion for about 10 minutes until it becomes soft and translucent

3. Turn off the heat, combine parsley and wine into a bowl, transfer the walnuts, apples, celery and onions into the saucepan and stir well.

4. Add the port mixture into the saucepan and set heat to medium, cook another 8-10 minutes until rice is done. Serve and enjoy!

# LUNCH

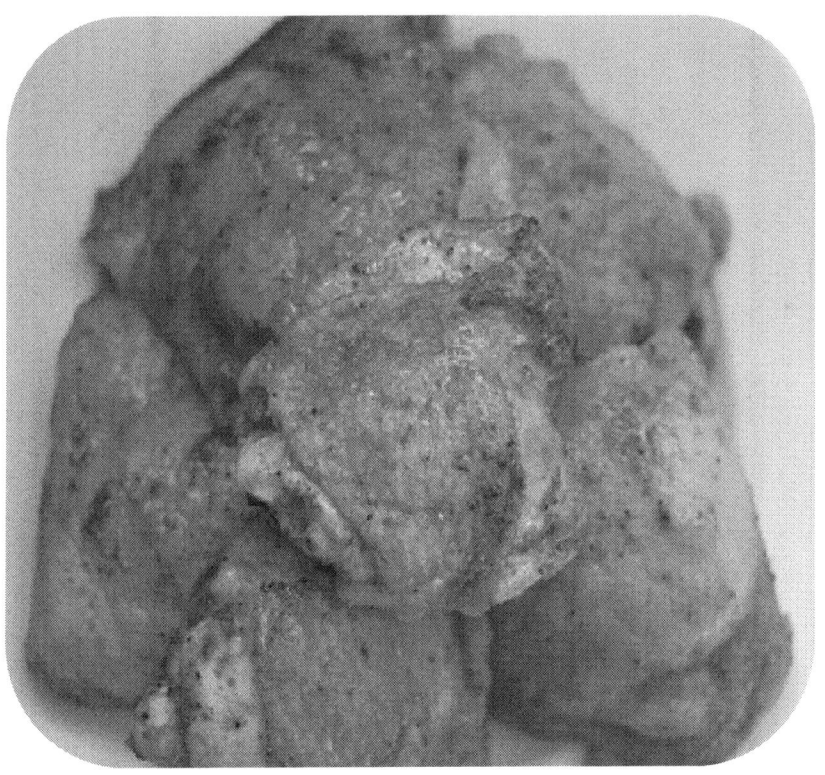

*Paprika Baked Chicken Thighs*

# Paprika Baked Chicken Thighs

Yields: 4 Serving

Preparation time: 10 minutes

Cooking time: 55 minutes

**Ingredients for Chicken Thighs:**

8 skinless chicken thighs

2 tablespoon of Spice Blend for Chicken

1/2 teaspoon of kosher salt

2 tablespoon of virgin olive

2 tablespoon of parsley, chopped

**Ingredients for Spice:** (Use 2 tablespoon for this recipe)

4 tablespoon of Smoked Paprika

3 tablespoon of Garlic Powder

1 tablespoon of Onion Powder

3 tablespoon of Ground Black Pepper

1 tsp Cayenne Pepper

3 tablespoon of Brown Sugar

**Instructions for Spice:**

1. Add all ingredients into a bowl or a jar with a lid and seal tightly, shake until well combined, set aside for later.

**Instructions for Chicken:**

1. Preheat oven to 450F

2. Next, transfer the chicken to a bowl, drizzle 2 tablespoons of spice, 2 tablespoons of oil and 1/2 teaspoon of kosher salt, mix and massage into the chicken

3. Add the chicken to the baking pan and bake for about 40 minutes or until preferred doneness. Enjoy!


## Mushroom and Leek Soup

Yields: 6 servings

Preparation time: 10 minutes

Cooking time: 30 minutes

Ingredients:

4 oz of sliced fresh mushrooms

1 cup leeks, sliced

2 tbsp of margarine

2 tablespoon of parsley, chopped

1/2 cup orzo pasta, uncooked

1/2 cup dry sherry

3 3/4 cups of water

3 10.5 oz cans of condensed beef broth

1/2 tsp Garlic Powder

2 tbsp of olive oil

1/2 tsp of ground black pepper

**Instructions:**

1. First, add the margarine into a large pot over low-medium heat, sauté the leeks and mushrooms until tender, stir in sherry and cook until the liquid reduces slightly.

2. Add the condensed beef broth, water and pepper. Bring to a boil and add the pasta. Boil gently for 10 minutes, or until the pasta is tender.

3. Serve with sliced mushrooms, enjoy!

## Smoked Salmon and Egg Salad

Yields: 8 servings

Preparation time: 5 minutes + 2 hours to refrigerate

**Ingredients:**

12 boiled eggs, peeled and chopped.

2 chopped celery stalks

1 red onion, chopped

5 oz of smoked salmon, diced

1 cup of mayonnaise

3 tbsp of fresh dill, chopped

Salt and pepper to taste

**Instructions:**

1. Combine the first 5 ingredients into a bowl with a lid

2. Season with salt, dill and pepper, taste to adjust seasoning as preferred

3. Refrigerate for about 2 hours, enjoy!

# Mandarin Orange Chicken Salad

Yields: 4 servings

Preparation time: 15 minutes

Cooking time: 10 minutes

**Ingredients:**

Olive oil

2 skinless boneless chicken breasts, chopped finely

2 tbsp of teriyaki sauce

2 tbsp of mandarin orange juice

Salt to taste

2 cups of mandarin oranges, drained juices

6 cups lettuce

**Instructions:**

1. Heat olive oil in a skillet over medium heat for 30 seconds, afterwards add the chicken and cook for 3 minutes until it browns.

2. Add teriyaki sauce and orange juice, cook for about 5 minutes and stir frequently, this enables the dressing to absorb fully into the chicken.

3. Place lettuce into a large sized bowl, add the chicken mixture, mandarin oranges, toss to combine.

4 Transfer to a plate and serve, enjoy!

# Very Berry Spinach Salad

Yields: 4 servings

Preparation time: 5 minutes

**Ingredients:**

1 6-ounce bag of baby spinach

1 cup cooked chicken breast, cubed

1 cup mixed berries - blackberries, raspberries, blueberries

1/2 cup sun dried tomatoes, chopped

1/2 cup of mushrooms, sliced

2 tbsp of balsamic vinegar

1/4 cup of roasted walnuts, chopped

2 tbsp of olive oil

1/2 tsp of kosher salt

**Instructions:**

1. Mix in the chicken, tomatoes, walnuts, mushrooms, spinach and berries in a large bowl

2. In a separate smaller bowl, stir in the salt, vinegar and oil, combine well and transfer to the larger bowl.

3. Transfer to a plate and serve, enjoy!

# Spiced Cauliflower With Peas

Yields: 2 Serving

Preparation time: 10 minutes

Cooking time: 30 minutes

**Ingredients:**

2 tbsp olive oil

1/2 teaspoon of mustard seeds

10 1/2 oz of cauliflower

1/2 teaspoon of turmeric powder

1/2 teaspoon of cumin seeds, crushed

1 teaspoon of fresh ginger, grated

3 small round chili

31/2 oz frozen peas

1 large tomato, chopped finely

3 teaspoon lime juice

Coriander leaves, chopped finely

Salt, white pepper to taste

**Instructions:**

1. Heat olive oil in a skillet over medium heat for 30 seconds, afterwards add mustard seeds and cook until it begins to pop.

2. Next, add the turmeric powder, cumin seeds, ginger and chili. Cook, stir frequently for 30 seconds.

3. Rinse and cut the cauliflower into little florets pieces, add to the spices and cook for about 5 minutes.

4. After that, reduce heat to low, add tomatoes, frozen peas, salt and pepper and cook for 20 minutes and cauliflower is ready

5. Transfer to a plate, served garnished with lime juice and coriander. Enjoy!

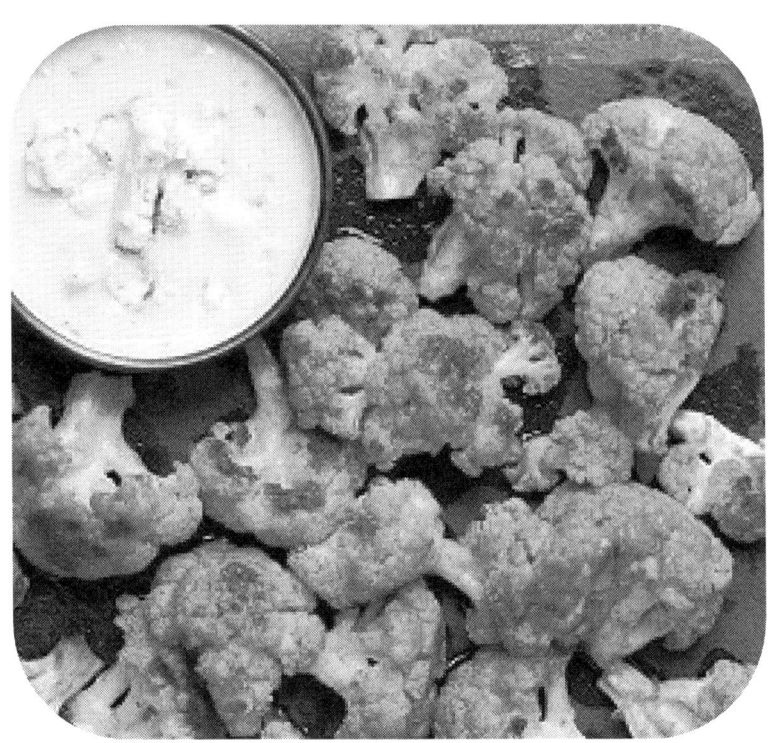

*Baked Buffalo Cauliflower Wings*

# Baked Buffalo Cauliflower Wings

Yields: 4 serving

Preparation time: 10 minutes

Cooking time: 40 minutes

**Ingredients:**

1 head of cauliflower, cut in 4 cups of florets

1/2 cup water

1/2 cup soy milk

3/4 cup gluten-free rice flour

1 teaspoon of cumin

1 teaspoon of paprika

1/4 tsp salt and ground pepper

2 teaspoon of garlic powder

1 tablespoon butter

1 cup red hot sauce

**Instructions:**

1. First preheat oven to 400F, evenly grease baking sheet with oil, set aside.

2. Rinse and cut cauliflower into little florets. With a medium sized bowl, combine the milk, flour, spices and water and stir until the mixture turns thick.

3. Fully dip the florets into the mixture, remove excess batter by shaking florets lightly, arrange in a single layer into the greased baking sheet and transfer to the oven.

4. Bake florets for 10 minutes, flip over and bake for another 10 minutes, this ensures that all sides turn golden brown

5. While florets bake, prepare buffalo wing sauce by placing the butter and hot sauce into a skillet on low heat, melt for about 30 seconds, stirring frequently. Remove from heat and transfer to a large sized bowl, set aside.

6. After 20 minutes, remove cauliflower from the oven into the large sized bowl containing the sauce, toss to enable florets coat evenly.

7. Return florets to the baking sheet and bake for about 10 minutes more. Serve, .if desired with preferred dipping sauce. Enjoy!


## White Bean Chili with Herbed Yogurt Cheese
Yields: 5 servings

Preparation time: 30 Minutes

Cooking time: 2 Hours

**Ingredients:**

3 cups of white beans, picked and rinsed

2 small poblano chili peppers

1 tbsp of butter, unsalted

4 cloves of minced garlic

1 onion, diced 1/4 inch

1 large carrot, diced 1/4-inch

2 stalks celery, diced 1/4-inche

1 tsp of cumin, ground

1 tsp of coriander, ground

1/2 tsp of paprika

30oz of low-sodium canned chicken stock

8 cups of water

1 1/2 teaspoons of salt

1/4 teaspoon of black pepper

4 grated radishes,

Cilantro sprigs, to garnish

Herbed Yogurt Cheese

**Instructions:**

1. Fill a large sized saucepan with about 3 inches of water. Place over high heat, add beans, bring to a strong boil, and set aside to stand for about an hour. After an hour drain the water from beans.

2. While the beans stands, place peppers into a medium baking sheet, transfer to the oven and roast, turning until both sides are evenly charred. Remove from oven, peel the charred skin,, remove ribs and seeds, discard them. Slice the pepper into 1/4-inch pieces, place in a small bowl and set aside.

3. Place a saucepan over low heat, add butter and heat until it melts ,increase heat to medium and add the diced onions, carrot, garlic and celery and cook for about 10-15 minutes until it becomes slightly browned, stir frequently.

4. Stir in the paprika, cumin and coriander. Add the water, chicken stock, beans and half the roasted pepper and cook covered for about an hour. Uncover and stir gently to make sure beans fall apart, add salt and pepper and cook for an extra 30 minutes

5. Serve garnished with grated radish, cilantro sprigs, poblano peppers, and yogurt cheese, enjoy.

# Mediterranean Roast Chicken

Yields: 5 servings

Preparation time: 20 minutes

Cooking time: 1 hour

**Ingredients:**

1 whole chicken

1/4 cup olive oil

1 large sized orange, juiced

1/4 cup Dijon mustard

4 tsp of Greek oregano, dried

Salt and freshly ground black pepper to taste

12 medium potatoes, peeled and diced

5 minced garlic cloves

**Instructions:**

1. Preheat oven to 375 F.

2. Add the mustard, olive oil, oregano, orange juice, salt, and pepper in a large bowl, stir to combine well. Place potatoes to the bowl and coat thoroughly, transfer to large sized baking sheet.

3. Place the garlic cloves under the skin of the chicken, place into the spice mixture and coat evenly and thoroughly, until all areas are covered.

4. Place chicken over potatoes, drizzle leftover mixture over and around the baking sheet and bake uncovered for about 80 minutes until juices run clear, check at 30 minutes intervals, add a small amount of warm/hot water if the potatoes look dry.

5. Remove baking sheet from the oven and transfer to a warm area, cover with aluminum foil and rest for about 15 minutes to enable retain moisture, Enjoy!

# Fish Tacos With Creamy Chipotle Sauce

Yields: 8 servings

Preparation time: 20 minutes

Cooking time: 1 hour

**Ingredients:**

**Tortillas:**

Canola oil

16 white corn tortillas

**Fish:**

1 tsp of garlic salt

1 tbsp of chile powder

Juice of 1 lime

2 tbsp of olive oil

1 1/2 pounds cod fish, diced into 4-ounce fillets

**Chipotle Sauce:**

2 tbsp of fresh cilantro, chopped

1 cup of mayonnaise

1 lime, juiced

1 tbsp of honey

2 canned chipotle chiles

A pinch of kosher salt

2 tbsp of olive oil

Purple cabbage, shredded

Fresh cilantro, for serving

Pico de Gallo:

2 ripe large tomatoes, diced finely

1 white onion, diced finely

1/2 minced jalapeno

1/2 bunch of fresh cilantro leaves, minced

1/2 lime, juiced

Kosher salt and freshly ground black pepper

**Instructions:**

1. In sets of 4, wrap tortillas in foil and place in an oven set to 325 F for 15 minutes until heated through and warm. Set aside

2. Next, add the garlic, chile powder, lime and all other ingredients for the fish into a large bowl, stir until well combined. Place the fish into the mixture and marinate for about 15 minutes.

3. Combine the first 6 ingredients of the chipotle sauce into a food processor and blend until smooth, transfer sauce to a container with a lid and set aside until ready to use.

4. Heat 2 tablespoons of olive oil in a skillet over medium heat for 30 seconds, add the fish and cook for 8 minutes, turning sides frequently until cooked through. Remove and transfer to a plate.

5. For the Pico de Gallo: Add all ingredients into a bowl and stir until well combined.

6. To make the tacos; add marinated fish fillets into 2 stacked tortillas, layer with the sauce, cilantro leaves, cabbage and the Pico de Gallo. Serve ,enjoy.

# Salmon with Pomegranate-Orange Relish

Yields: 4 servings

Preparation time: 15 minutes

Cooking time: 30 minutes

**Ingredients:**

2 medium carrots, chopped roughly

4 fresh skinless salmon fillets, an inch thick

¼ tsp of black pepper

½ tsp of salt

1/8 tsp of cayenne pepper

1 tbsp of butter

1 medium shallot, peeled and thinly sliced

2 medium oranges, peeled and sectioned

1 tbsp of honey

¼ cup of pomegranate seeds

**Instructions:**

1. Place carrots into a small saucepan containing a small amount of water, boil for about 5-10 minutes over medium-high heat until crisp and tender. Drain and set aside.

2. Rinse salmon with tap water and dry. Place on the unheated rack of a broiler pan, set aside.

3. Combine black pepper, salt and cayenne pepper into a small bowl, drizzle lightly and evenly over salmon fillets. Place salmon fillets 5 inches away from heat and roast for about 7 minutes

4. While the salmon cooks, heat butter in a large-sized skillet, add the carrots, shallots and cook over medium heat for 5 minutes until the shallots become slightly tender. Add oranges and cook for 1 minute, stir frequently. Add honey and stir. Remove from heat.

5. Serve with a layer of relish and salmon topped with a sprinkle of pomegranate seeds, enjoy.

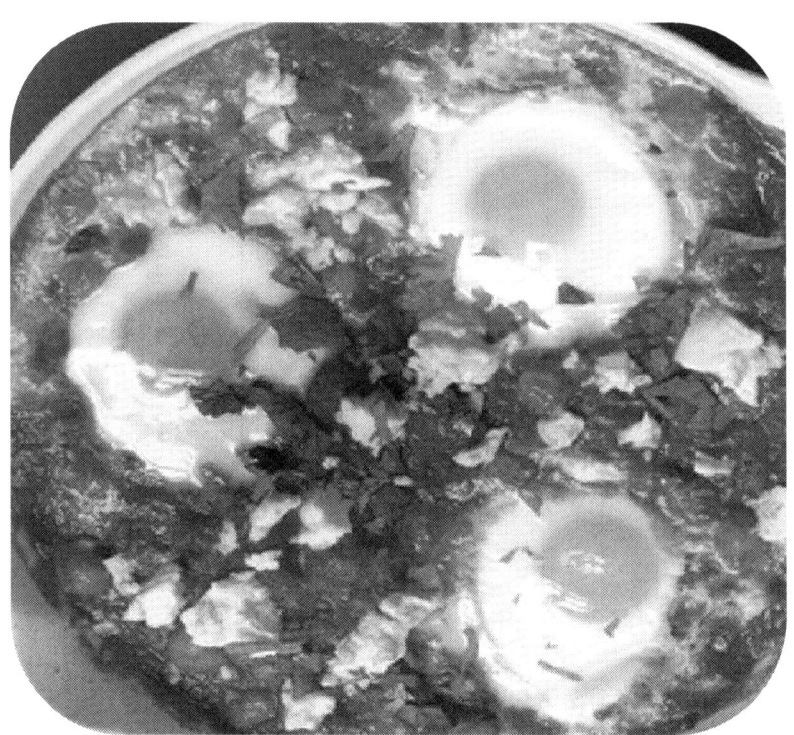

*Egg and Tomato Skillet with Pita (Shakshouka)*

# Egg and Tomato Skillet with Pita (Shakshouka)

Yields: 4 servings

Preparation time: 10 minutes

Cooking time: 35 minutes

**Ingredients:**

2 tbsp of olive oil

1 tsp of smoked paprika

2 cups of red sweet peppers, diced

½ cup onion, chopped

2 tbsp of no-salt tomato paste

2 tsp of red pepper, crushed

3 cups of tomatoes, chopped finely

1 tsp of ground cumin

¼ tsp of salt

4 large eggs

½ cup low-fat Greek yogurt

Snipped fresh parsley

2 whole-wheat pita bread rounds, halved crosswise

**Instructions:**

1. Heat olive oil in a large skillet set over medium heat, add the paprika, onion, tomato paste and red pepper, cook for 5 minutes until the onion becomes tender. Stir regularly.

2. Next stir in the cumin, tomatoes and salt. Reduce heat to low and simmer for about 10-15 minutes and the tomatoes break down.

3. After about 10 minutes, make 4 holes in the tomato mixture, break an egg and pour into the hole, repeat with the remaining eggs and cook on low heat for 5 minutes.

4. Add the Greek- yoghurt and a drizzle of parsley, serve with bread, enjoy!


## Italian-spiced Chicken and Mozzarella Melts
Yields: 8 servings

Preparation time: 15 minutes

Cooking time: 3 hours 40 minutes

**Ingredients:**

Nonstick cooking spray

8 skinless, boneless chicken thighs

2 medium-sized green sweet peppers, sliced thinly

½ tsp of dried rosemary, crushed

1 cup bottled spaghetti sauce

½ cup of pitted Kalamata olives, chopped roughly

1 cup of part-skim mozzarella cheese, shredded

¼ cup of fresh basil, snipped

2 tbsp of Parmesan cheese, grated

8 slices of whole grain Italian bread Apple slices

**Instructions:**

1. Coat a 4-quart slow cooker and a large-sized nonstick skillet lightly with the cooking spray

2. Place chicken in skillet over medium heat, cook until it turns golden brown on both sides.

3. Place pepper into the slow cooker, layer with chicken and a drizzle of rosemary. Add the spaghetti sauce and cook on high heat for 3 1/2 hours.

4. Preheat the broiler and afterwards, line a medium-sized baking sheet with aluminum foil. Set aside.

5. Place Chicken and pepper into a bowl, shred the chicken and add Kalamata olives, afterwards transfer cooking juices into a bowl, combine basil, parmesan and mozzarella cheese into a small bowl. Set aside.

6. Place bread on baking sheet and broil for 2 minutes about 5 inches away from heat until both sides are well toasted, top with the chicken and kalamata mixture, add a sprinkle of cooking juice and cheese mixture. Broil for 4 minutes until well toasted. Serve, enjoy!

# DINNER

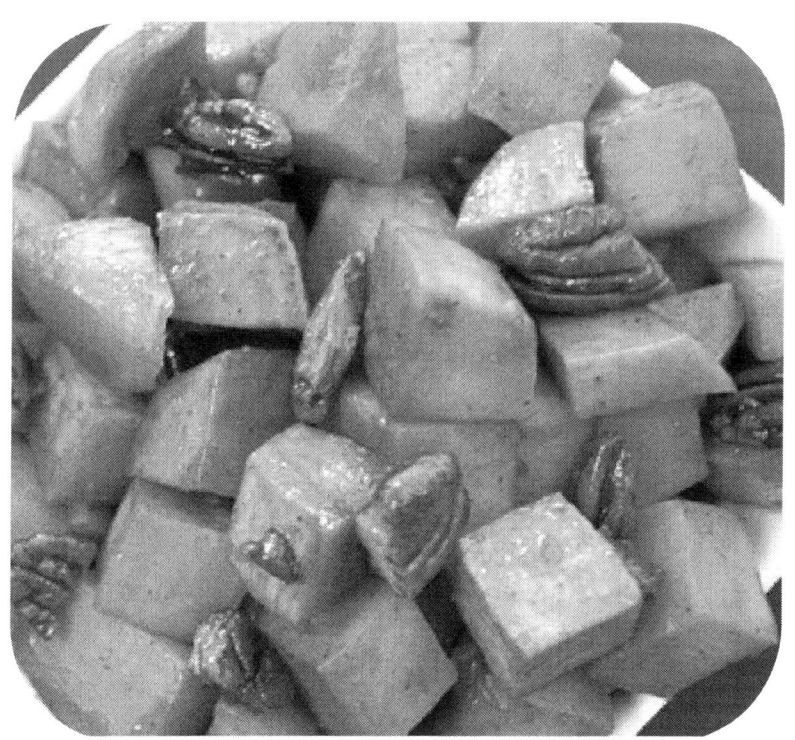

*Maple- Roasted Sweet Potatoes*

# Rice and Mushroom Casserole

Yields: 6 servings

Preparation time: 10 minutes

Cooking time: 35 minutes

**Ingredients:**

1 cup of long grain rice

4 tbsp of butter, divided

2 cups of fresh mushrooms, sliced

1 cup of onion, chopped

1 cup of celery, chopped

2 1/2 cups of water

2 beef bouillon cubes

1 can condensed mushroom soup if you want creamy rice

**Instructions:**

1. Preheat oven to 350F, spread 2 tablespoons of olive oil lightly but evenly into a medium sized casserole dish.

2. Brown the rice by placing into a saucepan set over low heat, stir constantly and cook for about 5minutes until the rice is completely brown, place 4 cups of water into a kettle and boil.

3. While the kettle boils, place the other 2 tablespoon of oil into a skillet set over low heat, add the mushrooms, onion and celery, cook until the mushroom loses its moisture and vegetables turns soft.

4. Next, pour 2 1/2 cups of boiled water into a bowl, add and dissolve the bouillon cubes, stir in the can of mushroom soup and transfer to the saucepan containing the  mushroom mixture to boil.

5. After it boils, lightly drizzle mushroom mixture into the casserole dish and bake for about 30 minutes until all liquid is absorbed, remove from the oven and stand for 10 minutes. Serve, enjoy!

# Maple- Roasted Sweet Potatoes

Yields: 12 servings

Preparation time: 10 minutes

Cooking time: 50 minutes

**Ingredients:**

1/3 cup of pure maple syrup

2 tbsp of butter, melted

1 tbsp of lemon juice

1/2 tsp of salt

Ground pepper

8 cups of sweet potatoes, peeled and cut into 1 1/2-inch

**Instructions:**

1. Preheat oven to 400F.

2. Combine all ingredients except the potatoes into a bowl and stir until well combined.

3. Set potatoes in an even layer over baking dish, drizzle maple syrup mixture over the potatoes and roast uncovered for 50 minutes. At 15 minutes intervals, stir potatoes until tender and slightly brown.

4. Remove from the oven and stand for 10 minutes. Serve, enjoy!

# Greek lamb meatballs with avocado goddess sauce

Yields: 4 servings

Preparation time: 20 minutes

Cooking time: 20 minutes

**Ingredients:**

1 pound ground lamb

2 cloves of garlic, minced

1 yellow onion, grated

2 tsp of cumin

1 tsp of dried oregano

1 lemon, zested

1/2 cup of fresh parsley, chopped

1/4 tsp of cayenne pepper

Kosher salt and black pepper

1 cup plain hummus

8 oz of feta cheese, cubed

arugula, tomatoes, Persian cucumbers, diced,

1 lemon, juiced

**Ingredients for the Avocado Sauce**

1 jalapeño, halved and seeded

1 avocado, halved

1/4 cup of plain Greek yogurt

1 cup of cilantro

1/2 cup of basil

2 lemons, juiced

1 tsp of cumin

Kosher salt

**Instructions:**

1. Preheat oven to 425 F, set a baking sheet with parchment paper.

2. Add the first 9 ingredients into a bowl and stir until combined well. Spread a bit of olive oil into your hands then roll the ground lamb into about 10 meatballs.

3. Transfer into the baking sheet and place into the oven to bake for 20 minutes until meatballs become cooked and slightly crisp.

4. To make the goddess sauce; Add all ingredients into a blender and blend until smooth, If the mixture turns out thick, add water a tablespoon at a time until mixture reaches desired consistency.

4. Serve by spreading the humus and avocado sauce into divided plates, add the meatballs, diced cucumber, tomatoes and arugula, Drizzle a tiny amount of olive oil and lemon juice. Enjoy!

# Hasselback Caprese Chicken

Yields: 4 servings

Preparation time: 10 minutes

Cooking time: 30 minutes

**Ingredients:**

Olive oil cooking spray

2 8oz boneless and skinless chicken breasts

½ tsp of salt, divided

½ tsp of ground pepper, divided

1 medium tomato, diced

3 oz of fresh mozzarella, halved and sliced

¼ cup prepared pesto

2 tbsp of olive oil

8 cups of broccoli florets

**Instructions:**

1. First preheat oven to 375F, afterwards lightly coat a large-sized baking sheet with cooking spray, set aside.

2. Season chicken with ¼ teaspoon of salt and pepper each, create crosswise slices almost to the bottom every 1/2 inch on both chicken breasts, fill opening with slices of mozzarella and diced tomato. Thoroughly brush with prepared pesto then place in a corner of the baking sheet.

3. Combine olive oil, broccoli, remaining salt and pepper into a bowl, stir in leftover tomato slices if any, after that place mixture in the empty area of the baking sheet.

4. Transfer baking sheet to preheated oven and bake for 20-25 minutes. Serve with broccoli, enjoy!

# Walnut-Rosemary Crusted Salmon

Yields: 4 servings

Preparation time: 10 minutes

Cooking time: 10 minutes

**Ingredients:**

Olive oil cooking spray

1 (1 pound) skinless salmon fillet, fresh

2 tsp of Dijon mustard

1 clove of minced garlic

¼ tsp of lemon zest

1 tsp of lemon juice

1 tsp of fresh rosemary, chopped

½ tsp of honey

½ tsp of kosher salt

¼ tsp of red pepper, crushed

3 tbsp of walnuts, finely chopped

3 tbsp of panko breadcrumbs

1 tsp of olive oil

**Instructions:**

1. First preheat oven to 425F.

2. Line a large-sized baking sheet with aluminum foil, coat with cooking spray and transfer salmon to the baking sheet, set aside.

3. With a small bowl, combine the first 8 ingredients (mustard-red pepper) in a bowl, combine the walnuts, olive oil and breadcrumbs in another bowl.

4. Coat salmon with the mustard mixture then drizzle walnut mixture, transfer to the oven and bake for 10 minutes until the fish flakes easily. Serve, enjoy!

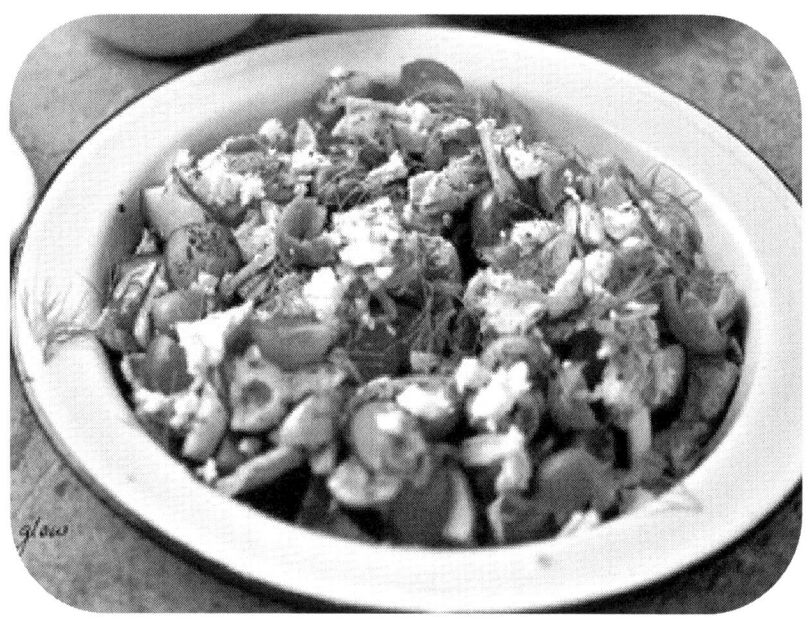

# Greek Salad Nachos

Yields: 6 servings

Preparation time: 10 minutes

**Ingredients:**

1 cup of prepared hummus

1 tbsp of lemon juice

2 tbsp of extra-virgin olive oil

¼ tsp of ground pepper

3 cups of whole-grain pita chips

½ cup of quartered grape tomatoes

2 tbsp of red onion, minced

2 tbsp of kalamata olives, chopped

¼ cup of crumbled feta cheese

1 cup of romaine lettuce, chopped

1 tbsp of fresh oregano, minced

**Instructions:**

1. Combine the first 4 ingredients into a small bowl

2. Spread the pita chips on a platter, top with ¾ of the hummus mixture then layer with the tomatoes, onion, olives, feta and lettuce.

3. Spread the remaining hummus and a drizzle of oregano. Serve, enjoy!

# Cod With Roasted Tomatoes

Yields: 4 servings

Preparation time: 10 minutes

Cooking time: 15 minutes

**Ingredients:**

4 fresh skinless cod fillets, ¾- to 1-inch thick

1 tsp of snipped fresh thyme

½ tsp of salt

¼ tsp of garlic powder

2 tsp of snipped fresh oregano

¼ tsp of paprika

¼ tsp of black pepper

Nonstick olive oil cooking spray

3 cups of cherry tomatoes

2 cloves of garlic, sliced

1 tbsp of olive oil

2 tbsp of pitted ripe olives, sliced

2 tsp of capers

Fresh oregano

**Instructions:**

1. Preheat oven to 450F. Line a large-sized baking sheet with aluminum foil and coat with cooking spray, set aside.

2. Add the thyme, salt, garlic powder, oregano, paprika and black pepper into a bowl, stir to combine well.

3. Rinse the fish, pat dry and drizzle half of the mixture on both sides until coated thoroughly and evenly. Transfer fish to one end of the baking sheet.

4. Place garlic and tomatoes on the other end of the baking sheet, Add olive oil to the remaining oregano mixture, stir to combine and after that spread mixture over the tomatoes and garlic.

5. Place baking sheet in the oven and bake for 10-12 minutes, check and stir tomatoes and garlic after 5 minutes.

6. Remove from oven and add capers and olives into the tomato and garlic mixture, stir to combine.

7. Serve fish with tomato and garlic mixture garnished with oregano, enjoy!

# Healthy Mediterranean Chicken With Orzo Salad

Yields: 4 servings

Preparation time: 15 minutes

Cooking time: 45 minutes

**Ingredients:**

2 skinless and boneless chicken breasts, halved

3 tbsp of extra-virgin olive oil, divided

1 tsp of lemon zest

½ tsp of salt, divided

½ tsp of ground pepper, divided

¾ cup whole-wheat orzo

2 cups baby spinach, sliced thinly

1 cup tomato, chopped

1 cup cucumber, chopped

2 tbsp of Kalamata olives, chopped

¼ cup crumbled feta cheese

¼ cup red onion, chopped

1 clove garlic, minced

2 tbsp of lemon juice

2 tsp of fresh oregano, chopped

**Instructions:**

1. Preheat oven to 425F. Line a large-sized baking sheet with aluminum foil, coat with cooking spray. Set aside.

2. Coat chicken with a tablespoon of olive oil, season with ¼ teaspoon of salt and pepper each and a light drizzle of lemon zest.

3. Transfer to prepared baking sheet and bake for 30 minutes. While it bakes, Add a quart of water to a medium saucepan set over medium-high heat and boil. Add wheat orzo and cool for 6 minutes, afterwards add the spinach and cook for 2 minutes more.

4. Drain liquid from the saucepan, rinse with cold water, drain and transfer to a bowl. Mix in tomato, cucumber, olives, feta cheese and onion to the bowl and set aside.

5. Add the remaining olive oil, garlic, lemon juice, oregano and salt and pepper into a bowl, stir to combine. Reserve a tablespoon of the mixture, combine the rest with the orzo mixture

6. Sprinkle the reserved dressing over the chicken, set aside for 10-15 minutes to enable flavor settle in. Serve with salad, enjoy!

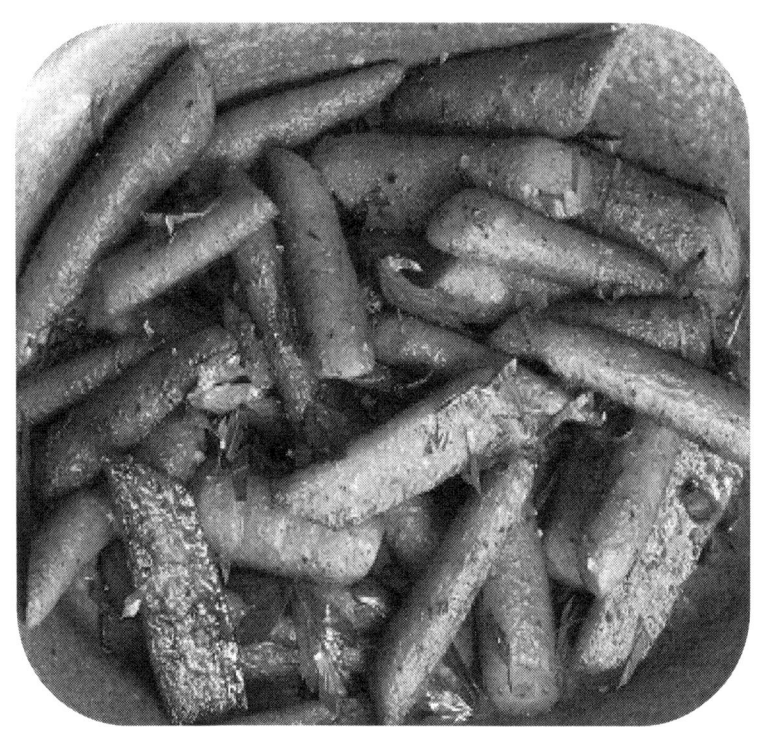

*Roasted Cumin Carrots*

## Roasted Cumin Carrots

Yields: 4 servings

Preparation time: 10 minutes

Cooking time: 20 minutes

**Ingredients:**

1 1/2 pounds of carrots, halved lengthwise

3 tbsp olive oil

1/4 cup pine nuts

1 orange

2 scallions, chopped

1/4 tsp ground cumin

Kosher salt and pepper

**Instructions:**

1. Preheat oven to 400F, coat the baking sheet with olive oil.

2. In a small bowl, combine the pine nuts and carrots, sprinkle with salt and pepper then spread in a single layer into the baking sheet and roast for about 15-20 minutes, or until the carrots become tender.

3. While the carrot roasts, peel off the skin and the pith of the orange, cut between the segment and a membrane using a sharp knife and set aside the membrane in a bowl.

4. Mix in the scallions, cumin and the remaining olive oil into the bowl until well combined.

5. Divide the roasted carrots into plates, top with orange mixture and serve. Enjoy!

# Healthy Chicken Dumpling Soup

Yields: 4 servings

Preparation time: 10 minutes

Cooking time: 35 minutes

**Ingredients:**

3 cups of water

1/2 tsp of salt

1/4 tsp of garlic powder

1 pound boneless skinless chicken breasts, cut into 1-1/2-inch pieces

3 cans (14-1/2 ounces each) reduced-sodium chicken broth

4 medium sized carrots, chopped

1 medium sized onion, chopped

1 celery rib, chopped

1 tsp of fresh parsley, chopped

1/4 tsp of chicken seasoning

1/4 tsp of pepper

**For the Dumplings:**

1/2 cup 1% cottage cheese

3 large sized egg whites

2 tbsp of water

1/4 tsp of salt

1 cup of flour

**Instructions:**

1. Place chicken breast into a large sized skillet over medium heat with cooking spray and cook the chicken for about 20 minutes or more, add the chicken broth seasoning and the vegetables .Cook uncovered for 20 minutes until the vegetables become tender.

2. For the Dumplings; Add cottage cheese and egg whites into a bowl, whisk until well combined then add the flour, water and salt. Whisk again to combine well

3. Reduce heat to low, drop dumplings into the skillet a tablespoon at a time. Cook covered for 15 minutes. Check for doneness by inserting a toothpick into dumplings. it should come out without crumbs. Enjoy!

## Red Lentil Chili

Yields: 4 servings

Preparation time: 10 minutes

Cooking time: 30 minutes

Ingredients:

1 onion, diced

6 cloves of minced garlic

1 red pepper, diced

4 tbsp of tomato paste

2 tsp of chili powder

2 tsp of dried oregano

2 bay leaves

2 tsp of ground cumin

3 tsp of smoked paprika

A can (780 g) diced tomatoes

A jar (570 g) of kidney beans, drained and rinsed

1 cup of red lentils, rinsed

1 cup of vegetable stock

2 tbsp of brown sugar

1 tsp of salt

Pepper, to taste

Lime slices

**Instructions:**

1. Pour a small amount of water into a saucepan set over medium heat, stir in the garlic and onion, sauté until soft. Add the red pepper and cook for 5 minutes.

2. Stir in the tomato paste, chili powder, oregano, bay leaves, cumin and paprika, cook for 30 seconds.

3. Set heat to low, add the diced tomatoes, beans, red lentils, vegetable stock and simmer for 20 minutes. Add more vegetable stock if little liquid remains.

4. Stir in the sugar, salt and pepper. Taste to adjust seasoning as desired. Cook for a few minutes then remove from heat.

5. Divide into plates and serve topped with fresh lime slices, enjoy!

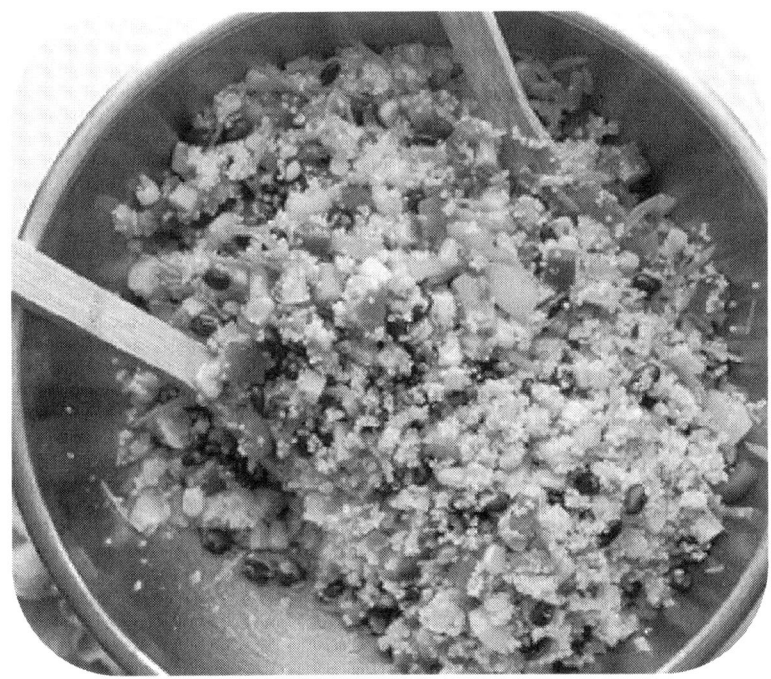

*Black Bean & Corn Quinoa*

Black Bean & Corn Quinoa

Yields: 4 servings

Preparation time: 10 minutes

Cooking time: 20 minutes

**Ingredients:**

2 tbsp of olive oil

1 medium sized sweet red pepper, chopped finely

1 medium sized onion, chopped finely

1 medium sized green pepper, chopped finely

2 tsp of chili powder

1/4 tsp of salt and pepper each

2 cups of vegetable stock/ chicken stock

1 cup of frozen corn

1 cup quinoa, rinsed

1 can (15 ounces) black beans, rinsed and drained

1/3 cup plus 2 tbsps fresh cilantro, minced and divided.

**Instructions:**

1. Place the olive oil and heat for 1 minute in a  large sized skillet over medium heat, add red pepper, onion and the green pepper, cook for 5 minutes, stir frequently.

2. Drizzle in the salt and pepper and cook until the vegetables are slightly tender.

3. Stir in the corn, quinoa and vegetable stock, reduce heat to low and cook for 15 minutes until the liquid evaporates.

4. Next, add beans and the 1/3 cup of cilantro, heat for 5 minutes, stir frequently, stir in reserved 2 tablespoon of cilantro and simmer. Enjoy!

# Healthy High Protein Chicken Parmesan Meatloaf Recipe

Yields: 4 servings

Preparation: 10 minutes

Cooking time: 45 minutes

**Ingredients:**

1 pound Ground Chicken Breast

1 Large Egg, beaten

1/3 cup Oats

¼ cup of Parmesan Cheese

½ cup Onion, diced

1 clove Garlic, minced

½ cup Pasta Sauce

3 ounce Mozzarella Cheese slices

2 tablespoon of Italian Seasoning

Salt & Pepper

**Instructions:**

1. Preheat oven to 375F, coat a medium sized baking sheet lightly but evenly with oil.

2. Next, add all ingredients including ¼ cup of pasta sauce into a bowl, stir to combine well

3. Knead flour into a loaf, place in baking sheet and bake for 40 minutes. Afterwards, remove from the oven and layer with the cheese and leftover pasta sauce.

4. Place in the oven and cook until cheese melts, remove and sit for 10-15 minutes before serving, enjoy!

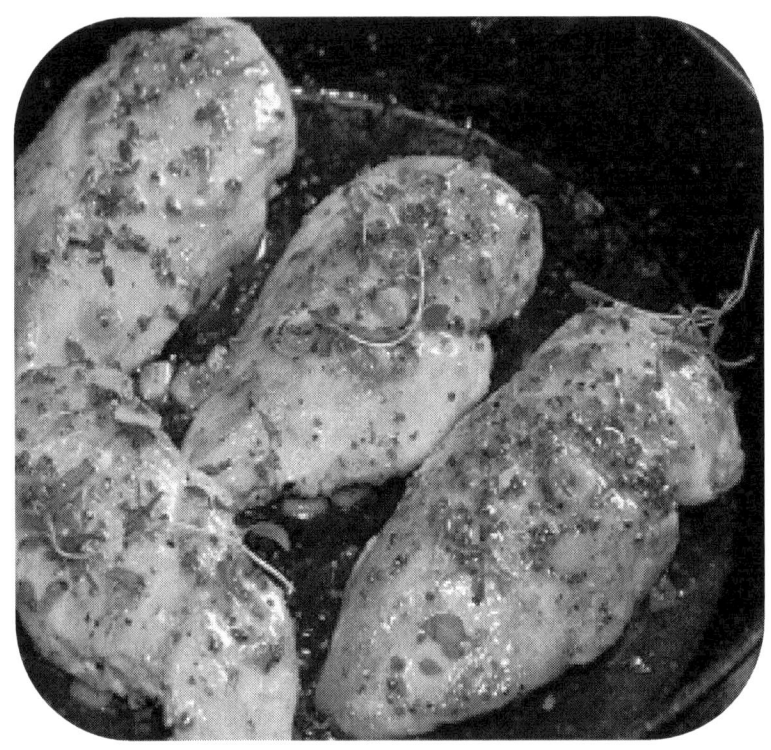

*Maple Mustard Glazed Chicken*

## Maple Mustard Glazed Chicken

Yields: 4 servings

Preparation time: 5 minutes

Cooking time: 20 minutes

**Ingredients:**

4 chicken breasts, boneless and skinless

2 tablespoons of olive oil

1/3 cup of Dijon mustard

1/3 cup of pure maple syrup

1 tbsp of apple cider vinegar

1 1/2 tsp of garlic, minced

1/4 tsp of salt

1/8 tsp of black pepper

**Instructions:**

1. In a large skillet set over medium-high heat, heat 2 tablespoon of olive oil, afterwards add the chicken breasts and cook until browned, set aside in a bowl and cover to retain heat.

2. Combine the remaining ingredients into a bowl. Transfer to the skillet and boil, reduce heat to low, add the chicken and simmer in the sauce for 5-7 minutes, Serve topped with herbs of your choice, enjoy!

# Chicken Provençal

Yields: 4 servings

Preparation time: 5 minutes

Cooking time: 20 minutes

**Ingredients:**

4 boneless, skinless chicken breast halves, trimmed, pounded to 1/2-inch thickness

1/4 cup of all-purpose flour

2 tbsp of vegetable oil

3 cloves of minced garlic

1/2 cup of white wine

1 15 ounce can of diced tomatoes, drained

1/3 cup of kalamata olives, pitted and chopped

1 tbsp of fresh parsley, chopped finely

Salt

**Instructions:**

1. Place flour into a bowl,

2. Lightly coat chicken breasts with salt, afterwards, dip into the bowl of flour and coat both sides

3. In a large skillet set over medium-high heat, heat the 2 tablespoon of oil, add the chicken breasts and cook until browned, set aside in a bowl and cover to retain heat.

4. Combine the remaining ingredients except the kalamata olive and parsley into a bowl. Place in the skillet and boil, set heat to low, add olives and simmer for 5 minutes.

5. Serve chicken with sauce topped with parsley, enjoy!

# Portobello Steaks With Lemon Basil Aioli

Yields: 4 steaks

Preparation time:

Cooking time:

**Ingredients:**

4 large Portobello, caps and stem removed

3 tbsp of olive oil

4 tbsp of balsamic vinegar

1 tbsp of soy sauce

1/2 tsp of dried oregano

3/4 cup plain yogurt

1 tsp of lemon zest + juice of 1/2 lemon

1/2 cup of fresh basil leaves

2 cloves of garlic

Salt to taste

**Instructions:**

1. Coat a cast iron skillet and preheat over low-medium heat, combine the ,oil, vinegar, oregano and a small pinch of salt and pepper into a bowl, coat portobello caps and marinade in the sauce for about 10 minutes.

2. To prepare the aioli; add the yogurt, lemon zest, juice, garlic and basil leaves into a blender, blend in bursts of 10 seconds until smooth, add salt. if thick, reduce consistency by adding water a tablespoon at a time.

3. Place the mushroom caps into the skillet and cook for about 8 minutes, flip on each sides at regular intervals until tender. Serve with aioli, enjoy!

# DESSERT

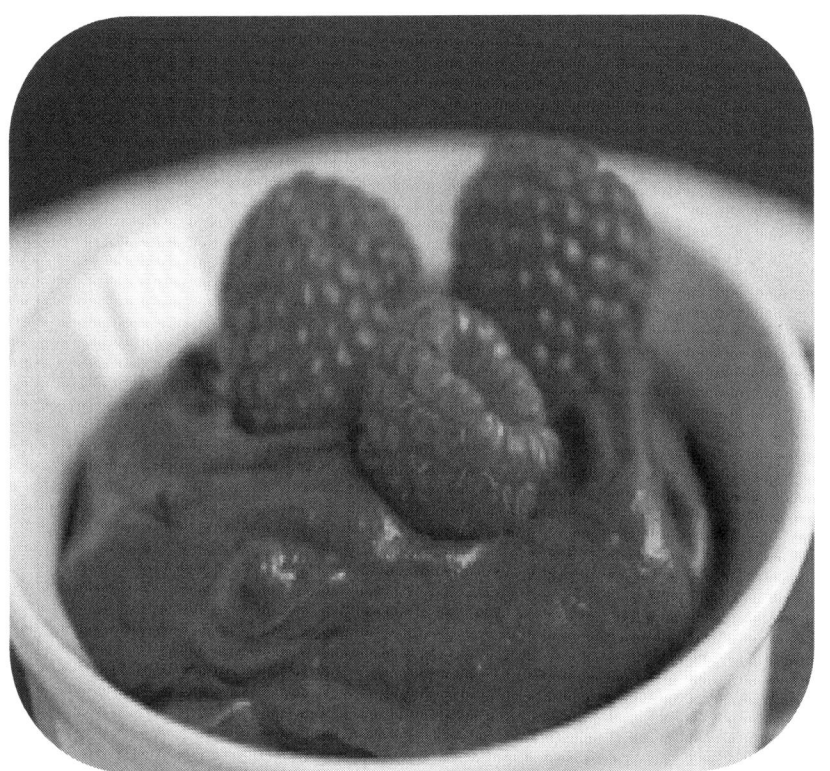

# Raspberry -Pineapple Parfaits

Yields: 4 servings

Preparation time: 5 minutes

**Ingredients:**

16 oz of peach nonfat yogurt

1/2 pint of raspberries

1 1/2 cup of pineapple chunks

**Instructions:**

1. Layer raspberries, pineapples and yogurt into 4 glasses. Serve, enjoy!

Avocado Chocolate Mousse`

Yields: 4 servings

Preparation time: 10 minutes + 30 minutes chill time

**Ingredients:**

2 ripe avocados, halved

1/3 cup of honey

1/3 cup of cocoa powder, unsweetened

2 tablespoon of unsweetened almond milk

1/2 teaspoon of vanilla extract

1/2 teaspoon of chia powder

1/8 teaspoon of kosher salt

Fresh raspberries to garnish

**Instructions:**

1. Add honey, cocoa powder, almond milk, vanilla extract, chia powder and kosher salt into a bowl. Scoop the flesh from the avocado and place in the bowl.

2. Combine all ingredients into a blender and blend until smooth, spoon into a bowl and refrigerate for about 30 minutes-1 hour. Serve garnished with raspberries. Enjoy!

Salted Caramel Coconut Bliss Balls
Yields: 12 balls

Preparation time: 15 minutes + 1 hour chill time

**Ingredients:**

1 cup almonds

1 cup pitted Medjool dates

1/4 cup of unsweetened shredded coconut + extra

1/4 tsp salt

**Instructions:**

1. Combine all ingredients into a food processor, pulse until it turns into a sticky paste.

2. Place on a flat surface and shape into bite sized balls. Lightly drizzle with shredded coconut and roll to coat. Transfer into an airtight container and refrigerate for an hour before serving. Enjoy!

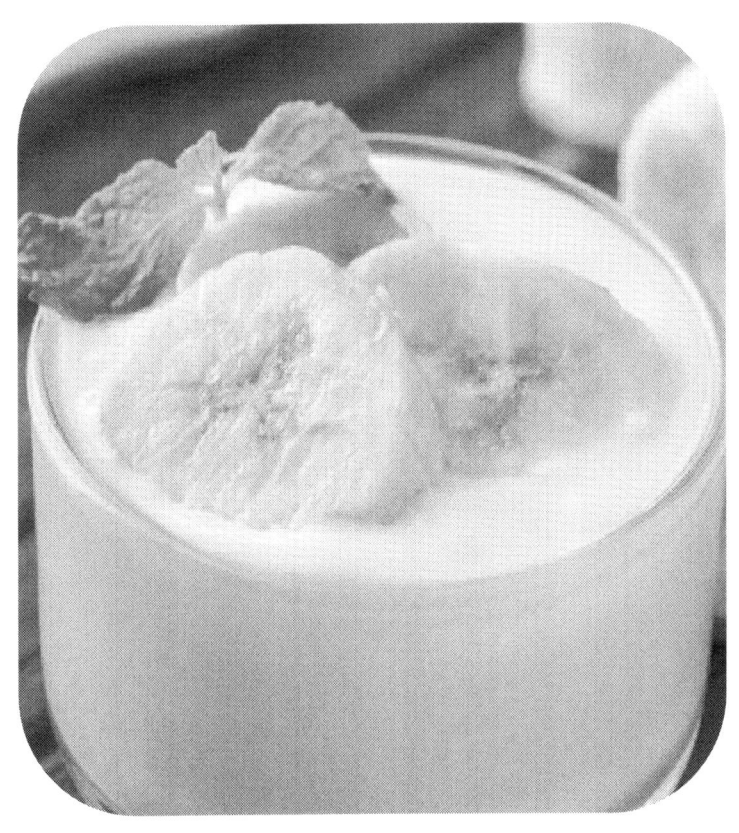

*Banana Custard Pudding*

# Banana Custard Pudding

Yields: 4 servings

Preparation time: 10 minutes

Cooking time: 15 minutes + 1 hour chill time

**Ingredients:**

1/2 tbsp of cornstarch

1/3 cup of sugar

1/8 tsp of salt

1-1/2 cups of almond milk

3 egg yolks, beaten

1 tsp of vanilla extract

1 medium-sized banana, sliced

Fresh mint, optional

**Instructions:**

1. Combine the first 3 ingredients into a saucepan set over medium heat, add milk and stir until smooth. Cook until it turns thick and bubbly stirring regularly. Reduce heat to low.

2. Add a small amount of filling into the egg, stir then combine with ingredients in the pan.

3. Increase heat to medium and boil, stir regularly. After 2 minutes, remove from heat and stir in vanilla.

4. Transfer to an airtight bowl and refrigerate for about an hour, Garnish with mint and  bananas before serving, enjoy!

# Apple Crisp

Yields: 12 servings

Preparation time: 10 minutes

Cooking time: 45 minutes

**Ingredients:**

10 cups of apples, peeled, cored and sliced

1 tbsp of flour

1 cup white sugar

1 tsp of ground cinnamon

1/2 cup of water

1 cup of quick-cooking oats

1 cup packed brown sugar

1/2 cup melted butter

1/4 tsp of baking powder

1 cup of all-purpose flour

1/4 tsp of baking soda

**Instructions:**

1. Preheat oven to 350F

2. Combine the flour, sugar and cinnamon in a small bowl, set aside.

3. Place sliced apples in a baking sheet, sprinkle cinnamon mixture and add 1/2 cup of water.

4. Combine the rest of the ingredients into a bowl, stir until well emulsified, spread evenly in the baking sheet.

5. Place in the oven and bake for 45 minutes. Enjoy!

# Sugar-free chickpea fudge

Yields: 4 servings

Preparation time: 15 minutes + 1 hour chill time

Cooking time: 30 minutes

**Ingredients:**

Chickpea fudge layer:

1 tin of chickpeas, cooked and drained

1/4 cup natural peanut butter

1 teaspoon of cinnamon'

1/4 cup honey

1 teaspoon of vanilla extract

1/4 cup + 1 tablespoon of coconut milk

2 tablespoon of coconut oil

**For the Chocolate Layer:**

5 tablespoon of coconut oil

2 tablespoon of honey

2 tablespoon of cocoa powder

Pinch of salt

**Instructions:**

1. Line a 26 cm x 16cm dish with cling wrap, set aside.

2. Remove the skin from the chickpeas by soaking in warm water for about 10 minutes, drain and cover in a kitchen towel and rub until the skin falls off

3. Combine the chickpea, peanut butter, cinnamon, honey, vanilla extract and coconut milk into a bowl, place in a food processor and blend until it

forms a smooth paste. Transfer to an airtight container and refrigerate for about 2 hours

**For the chocolate layer**

4. Combine all ingredients into a bowl and whisk until smooth. Pour over chilled chickpea fudge and refrigerate for 20 minutes

5. Cut into bite size chunks and serve, enjoy!

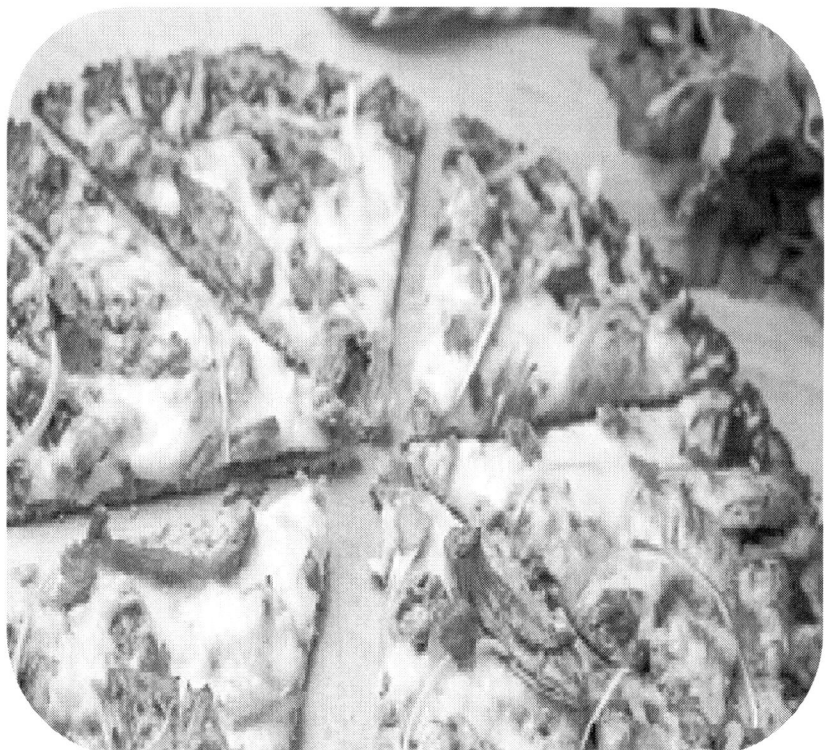

*Cauliflower Pizza Crust*

81

# Cauliflower Pizza Crust

Yields: 6 slices

Preparation time: 30 minutes

Cooking time: 30 minutes

**Ingredients:**

4 cups of cauliflower florets

2 1/2 tablespoon of chia seeds

1/4 cup water

1/3 cup almond flour

1 teaspoon of dried oregano

1/4 teaspoon of garlic powder

1/2 teaspoon of salt

**Instructions:**

1. First preheat oven to 450 F, line a baking sheet with aluminum foil, combine chia seeds and water into a bowl and refrigerate for 30 minutes.

2. Place florets into boiled water and steam until soft, drain water and squeeze out moisture by placing in a dish cloth, squeeze until as dry as possible. Mix with chia seed mixture and mash, set aside

3. Mix almond flour with oregano, garlic powder and salt in a medium sized bowl, combine with the chia mixture, shape into a ball and transfer to the baking sheet.

4. Use a rolling pin to flatten and spread the ball into a 1/4 inch thick circle. Transfer to the oven and bake for 20 minutes until it slightly turns brown with crisp edges.

5. Remove from oven and add toppings of your choice, bake for an extra 5 minutes. Enjoy!

# Dark chocolate coconut bites

Yields: 18

Preparation time: 10 minutes

Cooking time: 20 minutes

**Ingredients:**

2 cups of coconut, desiccated

4 tbsp of honey

5 tbsp of coconut oil

1 tsp of vanilla

4 oz of dark chocolate or chocolate chips for melting

**Instructions:**

1. Combine the honey, coconut oil and vanilla into a bowl.

2. Place the coconut into a blender and blend until smooth and thick, transfer to the bowl and stir until well combined.

3. Shape coconut paste by squeezing and gently shaping into a ball with your palm. Next, place balls in the refrigerator to chill until firm, this may take up to 30 minutes.

4. Melt the chocolate with an oven or microwave. Lay out a sheet of aluminum foil then coat the coconut balls by rolling with a fork into the bowl of melted chocolate, hold above the bowl to enable excess chocolate drip off.

5. Place coated chocolate on aluminum foil to enable chocolate harden, after it hardens, transfer to an airtight bowl and refrigerate for about an hour, enjoy!

## Dark Chocolate Black Bean Protein Brownies
Yields: 8

Preparation time: minutes

Cooking time: minutes

**Ingredients:**

1 can of black beans

¼ cup chocolate protein powder

1/2 ripe avocado

2 eggs, beaten

6 dates, pitted

¼ teaspoon of baking soda

½ teaspoon of baking powder

½ teaspoon of vanilla

½ teaspoon of salt

¼ cup of cocoa powder

1/4 cup cacao nibs

**Instructions:**

1. First, preheat oven to 350F. Lightly grease a medium sized baking sheet with olive oil.

2. Add all ingredients except cacao nibs into a blender and blend in bursts of 10 seconds until smooth. Add nibs and blend.

3. Transfer mixture to the baking sheet and spread evenly, bake for 20 minute.

4. Store in an airtight container and refrigerate for 30 minutes, enjoy!

# SOUP

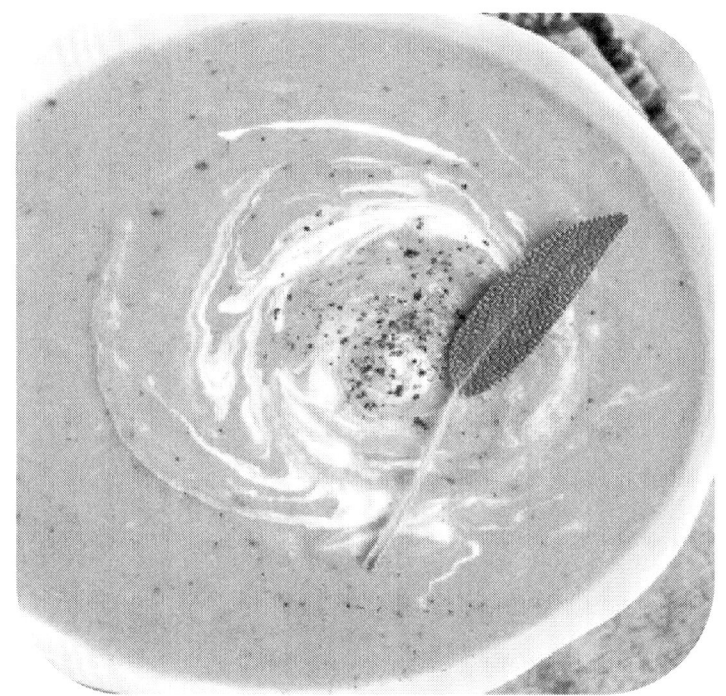

*Butternut and Granny Smith Apple Soup*

# Liver Cleanse Soup

Yields: 4 servings

Preparation time: 10 minutes

Cooking time: 1 hour

**Ingredients:**

3 cups of water

1 cup of organic vegetable broth

2 beets, diced

2 carrots, diced

2 broccoli, diced

10 clove of garlic, crushed

1 onion, diced

1/2 lemon, squeezed freshly

2 bay leaves

1/2 tsp of Himalayan pink salt

1/2 tsp of ground turmeric

1/2 tsp of ground oregano

1/2 tsp of freshly ground black pepper

**Instructions:**

1. Place all ingredients into a medium sized saucepan set over medium – high heat and bring to a boil.

2. Afterwards, reduce heat to low and simmer for about 40 minutes until vegetables become soft. Stir regularly.

3. Taste, adjust seasoning if needed and simmer for a little while, enjoy!

# Butternut and Granny Smith Apple Soup

Yields: 6 servings

Preparation time: 5 minutes

Cooking time: 35 minutes

**Ingredients:**

2 tbsp of unsalted butter

1 cup of leeks, diced

1 medium sized onion, diced

2 granny smith apples, cored, peeled and chopped

2 pounds of butternut squash, peeled and cubed

6 cups of chicken stock

Nutmeg to taste

Salt and pepper to taste

**For the Mascarpone Topping:**

1/2 cup of mascarpone cheese

1/2 tsp of cinnamon

2 tbsp of almond milk

**Instructions:**

1. Add butter to a large saucepan set over medium heat and melt

2. Add the leeks, onion and apples and sauté for 7 minutes until it becomes soft and translucent, next add the butternut squash and chicken stock. Reduce heat to low and simmer for 20 minutes until squash become tender.

3. While the soup simmers, to make the mascarpone topping; combine all ingredients into a bowl, stir to combine well, set aside.

4. Remove the soup from heat, set aside to cool for a few minutes. Transfer to a blender and blend until smooth.

5. Return soup to saucepan, stir in seasonings and simmer for 5 minutes over low heat, serve topped with mascarpone topping, enjoy!

## Tuscan White Bean Stew with croutons

Yields: 6 serving

Preparation time: 30 minutes

Cooking time: 45 minutes

**Ingredients:**

2 cups cannellini beans soaked overnight, rinsed and drained

6 cups water

1 bay leaf

1 tsp of salt

2 tbsp of olive oil

1 yellow onion, diced

3 carrots, peeled and chopped roughly

6 cloves of garlic, minced finely

¼ tsp of ground black pepper

1 tbsp of fresh rosemary, chopped

1½ cups vegetable stock

**For the Croutons**

1 tbsp of extra-virgin olive oil

2 cloves garlic, quartered

1 slice of whole-grain bread, cut into ½-inch cubes

**Instructions:**

For the Crouton:

1. Place olive oil in a large skillet over medium heat and heat.

2. Add garlic and sauté for 2 minutes until it becomes soft, remove from heat and set aside for 10 minutes. This enables the oil soak up the garlic.

3. Dispose the garlic, return skillet to medium heat and add the whole grain bread. Sauté for about 5 minutes until it turns light brown. Stir frequently.

4. Transfer to a bowl and set aside.

**For the Stew:**

1. Add the first 4 ingredients into a large saucepan set over medium-high heat, boil for 10 minutes. Reduce heat to low and cook for about an hour until the beans are tender.

2. Remove bay leaves, place 1/2 cup of beans liquid into a bowl, drain the rest and transfer beans to a bowl, set aside. Add 1/2 cup of beans into the bowl containing reserved liquid, mash until it forms a paste.

3. Set sauce pan over medium heat; heat olive oil, stir in carrot and onions and sauté for 6 minutes until the carrots are tender.

4. After that, add the garlic and cook for 1 minute until soft. Next add the salt, pepper, beans and beans paste, rosemary and vegetable stock into the pot, simmer for 5-10 minutes until cooked through.

5. Serve topped with croutons, enjoy!

# Lentil, Kale and Potato Soup

Yields: 4 servings

Preparation time: 10 minutes

Cooking time: 40 minutes

**Ingredients:**

1 tablespoon of olive oil

2 stalks of celery, chopped

1 medium sized onion, chopped

2 large sized carrots, chopped

4 cups of vegetables broth + 1/2 cup water

1 cup of lentils, rinsed and picked over (not red)

1 teaspoon of salt

1/2 teaspoon of garlic powder

1/4 teaspoon of cumin

1/4 teaspoon of coriander

1 1/2 cups diced potato

1/2 bunch of kale, ribs removed,  chopped

2 teaspoon of red wine vinegar

Salt and pepper, to taste

**Instructions:**

1. Heat olive oil in a large saucepan set over medium heat.

2. Add the celery, onions and carrots and cook for 7 minutes until it becomes soft and translucent.

3. Afterwards, add vegetable broth, water, lentils, garlic powder and cumin, coriander and salt, bring to a boil. Reduce heat to low and cook covered for 20 minutes.

4. Next add potatoes and cook until the potatoes are tender, this takes about 20 minutes, add kale and cook for 5 minutes. Remove from heat and add vinegar. Season with salt and pepper, serve, enjoy!


## Mediterranean Chicken Soup

Yields: 8 servings

Preparation time: 10 minutes

Cooking time: 25 minutes

**Ingredients:**

1-1/2 pounds of boneless and skinless chicken breasts cut in 3/4-inch

1 tbsp of Greek seasoning

1 tsp of freshly ground pepper

1 tbsp of olive oil

1 garlic clove, minced

4 green onions, sliced thinly

7 cups of reduced-sodium chicken broth

1/4 cup of white wine

1/4 cup sun-dried tomatoes, chopped and not packed in oil

1/4 cup pitted Greek olives, sliced

1 tbsp of capers, drained

1-1/2 tsp of fresh basil, minced

1-1/2 tsp of fresh oregano, minced

1-1/2 cups of uncooked orzo pasta

2 tbsp of lemon juice

1-1/2 tsp of fresh parsley, minced

**Instructions:**

1. Combine Greek seasoning and pepper in a small bowl, season chicken with mixture.

2. Place oil into a medium sized saucepan over medium heat, add chicken breasts and sauté until no longer pink, stir regularly. Remove chicken and set aside.

3. Stir in garlic and green onions and sauté for a minute, add white wine, stir.

4. Next, add the tomatoes, olives, broth and capers, oregano and basil and chicken, cover and bring to a boil.

5. Reduce heat to low and simmer for 10 minutes, mix in orzo and cook until pasta becomes tender. Stir in the Parsley and lemon juice and cook for 5 minutes. stir frequently.

6. Transfer to a bowl and serve, enjoy!

# Butternut Squash Apple Soup

Yields: 5 servings

Preparation time: 15 minutes

Cooking time: 1 hour

**Ingredients:**

2 1/2 cups of butternut squash, peeled & chopped, seeds removed

1 large sized carrots, peeled & chopped

1/2 medium sized sweet potato, peeled & chopped

1 medium sized granny smith apples, cored & chopped

1 medium sized potatoes, peeled & chopped

1/2 medium sized onion, peeled & chopped

5 cloves of minced garlic

1/2 celery stalks, chopped

5 tbsp of butter, divided

1/2 tbsp of extra virgin olive oil

2 cups of vegetable stock

3/4 cup of almond milk

1/2 cup of yogurt

salt and freshly ground black pepper

3 cooked and crumbled bacon pieces

Parsley, to garnish

**Instructions:**

1. Preheat oven to 350 F

2. Combine the first 5 ingredients, half the onion into a large casserole dish, drizzle in salt and pepper to season.

3. Spread 2 tablespoon of butter over vegetables, cover dish with aluminum foil and place into the oven to bake for 40 minutes, remove the aluminum foil and bake for 10 more minutes

4. Heat olive oil in a medium sized saucepan placed over low heat. Add the remaining onion and garlic and cook for a few minutes, stir regularly. Next add the butter, vegetable stock and cooked vegetables. Mash vegetables (with a handheld mixer). Increase heat to medium and cook for 10 minutes, stir frequently.

5. Transfer a cup of soup into a small bowl, add yoghurt and stir, set aside.

6. Pour almond milk into the soup and cook for 5 minutes, add yoghurt mixture and stir for a few seconds to incorporate well. Season with salt and pepper, taste to adjust seasoning as desired. Serve garnished with parsley and bacon. Enjoy!

## Detox Soup
Yields: 4 servings

Preparation time: 15 minutes + 30 minutes

Cooking time: 15 minutes

**Ingredients:**

1 tbsp of olive oil

½ cup yellow onion, chopped

2 cups of broccoli florets

1 ripe avocado, chopped

2 cups of arugula

1 tsp of lemon juice + zest

2 cups low-sodium vegetable stock

**Instructions:**

1. Heat olive oil in a large sized saucepan placed over low heat. Add the remaining onion and cook for a few minute until soft, stir regularly.

2. Increase heat to medium; add the vegetable stock and boil, as the water begins to boil, add the broccoli and cook covered for 5 minutes stir at 1 minute intervals.

3. Remove soup from heat and cool for 30 minutes. Add the avocado, arugula and the lemon juice and puree in a blender.

4. Reheat before serving, serve with a pinch of lemon zest, enjoy!


## Creamy Vegan Red Lentil and Kale Soup
Yields: 4 servings

Preparation time: 10 minutes

Cooking time: 30 minutes

**Ingredients:**

1 1/2 cups red lentils, uncooked

3 cups of vegetable broth

2 cups of tomatoes, chopped

1/2 onion, chopped

1 tsp of Himalayan pink salt

2 tbsp of tomato sauce

1 1/2 tsp of ground cumin

1-2 pinch of cayenne pepper

**Add-ins:**

1 cup of kale, destemmed and chopped

1 can of coconut milk, 13.5 oz

**Instructions:**

1. Combine all soup ingredients into a medium sized saucepan over medium heat, stir and bring to a boil

2. Set heat to low and cook covered until the lentils become soft, this takes about 25 minutes, stir regularly. Add kale and coconut milk, stir and cook for 2 minutes, remove from heat and serve, enjoy!


## Ginger and Carrot Soup
Yields: 6 servings

Preparation time: 10 minutes + 3 hours chill time

Cooking time: 40 minutes

**Ingredients:**

2 tbsp of olive oil

1 medium sized onion, chopped

1 2-inch piece of fresh ginger, peeled and grated

1 clove garlic, chopped

10-12 carrots, chopped

6 cups of low-sodium vegetable broth

1 lime, juiced + plus lime wedges to garnish

1 cup plain nonfat yogurt

Salt and freshly ground black pepper

**Instructions:**

1. Heat oil into a medium sized saucepan over low heat, sauté onion until soft and translucent, add in the ginger and garlic and sauté for 1 minute.

2. Next, increase heat to medium, add carrots and vegetable broth, cook covered for 5 minutes. Set heat to low and simmer for about 25 minutes until carrots become tender. Remove from heat and cool.

3. Place soup in a blender and blend until smooth, transfer to a bowl with a lid and refrigerate for about 3 hours until chilled.

4. Remove from fridge, Add the yogurt and lime juice, salt and pepper and stir, taste to adjust seasoning as desired. Serve garnished with lime wedges, enjoy!

# SALAD

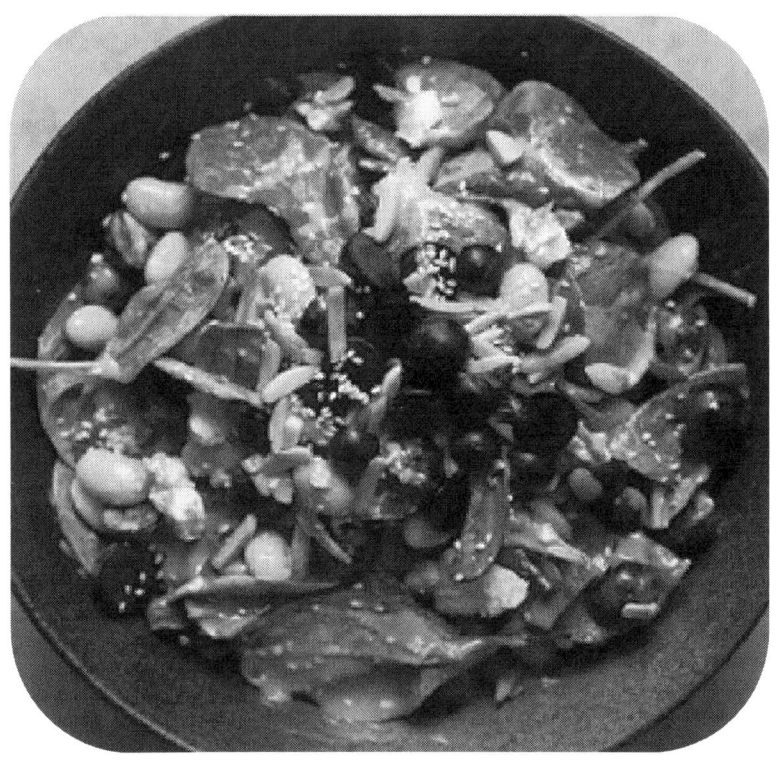

## Carrot-Ginger Salad

Yields: 4 servings

Preparation time: 20 minutes + 30 minutes to refrigerate

**Ingredients:**

**For the Salad:**

1/2 cup of golden raisins

1/2 cup of cranberries, dried

1/2 cup of slivered almonds

5 medium sized carrots, shredded

**For the Dressing:**

1/3 cup white vinegar

2 tbsp of ginger, grated

2 tbsp of cilantro, chopped finely

2 tsp of salt

1/2 tsp of pepper

1 tsp of sugar

1/2 cup of canola oil

**Instructions:**

For the Salad:

1. Add almonds to a skillet over low-medium heat and cook for about 10 minutes until it turns golden brown. While the almond cooks, place a small saucepan filled with water on another burner to boil. Transfer almonds to a bowl and set aside.

2. Add the cranberries and raisins into a small bowl, pour the boiling water and soak for 10 minutes, afterwards drain the water and transfer contents to a separate bowl, add the carrots.

**For the Dressing:**

1. Mix all the ingredients into a large bowl, stir until properly combined, then add the bowl of carrot mixture and toss to coat evenly.

2. Refrigerate for about 30 minutes, add in almonds and serve, enjoy!


## Healthy Shamrock Shake Recipe

Yields: 2 large cups

Preparation time: 5 minutes

**Ingredients:**

2 cups of soy milk

1 teaspoon of mint extract

2 teaspoon of vanilla extract

4 cups of ice cubes

½ avocado peeled

¼ cup of raw honey

1 cup raw spinach

**Instructions:**

1. Add all ingredients apart from the ice cubes into a blender and blend until smooth, add the ice cubes and blend some more.

2. Transfer contents into cups, enjoy!

# Kale and Apple Salad

Yields: 3 servings

Preparation time: 20 minutes

**Ingredients:**

3 tbsp of fresh lemon juice

1/4 teaspoon kosher salt

2 tbsp of extra-virgin olive oil

1 bunch kale, ribs removed, sliced thinly

1/4 cup dates, sliced thinly

1 Honeycrisp apple, sliced thinly

1/4 cup of toasted slivered almonds,

1/4 cup of Pecorino, grated finely

Ground black pepper

**Instructions:**

1. First, add the olive oil, lemon and salt into a bowl, stir to combine well.

2. Add kale and toss, stand for about 10 minutes then add the almond, apples, dates and cheese. Season with the pepper or additional salt as required, toss once more and serve, enjoy!

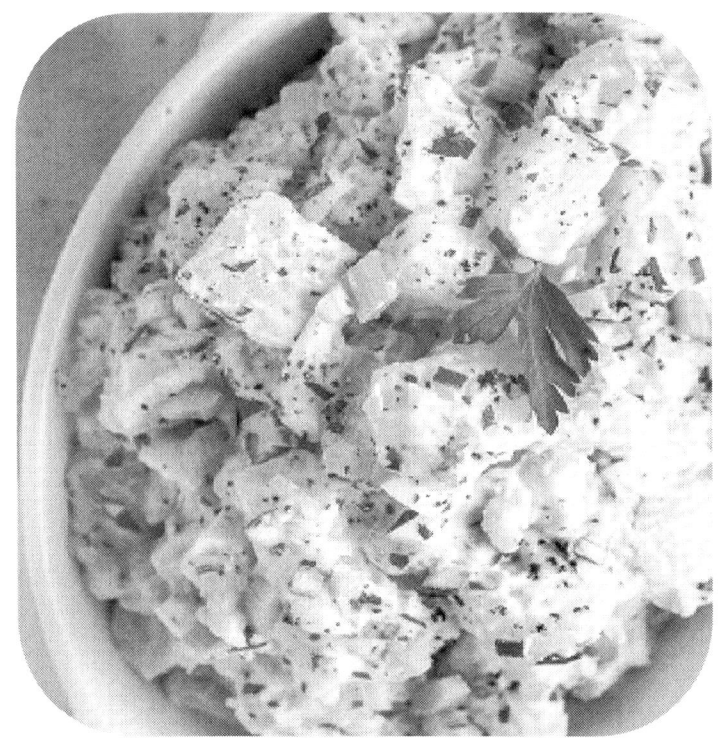

*Potato Salad Recipe*

## Classic Potato Salad Recipe

Yields: 4 servings

Preparation time: 10 minutes

Cooking time: 20 minutes

Ingredients:

2lbs of Yukon Gold potatoes, peeled and diced into 1-inch pieces

2 tsp of Dijon mustard

3/4 cup sour cream

1/4 cup mayonnaise

1 tbsp of fresh lemon juice

1/2 cup celery, chopped

1/4 cup parsley, chopped

1/2 cup of green onions, sliced thinly

3/4 cup of dilli pickles, chopped into 1/4 in cubes

Salt

Freshly ground pepper

**Instructions:**

1. Place potatoes into a saucepan placed over medium heat, filled with water. Add a pinch of salt and bring to a boil, reduce heat and simmer for about 10 minutes until the potatoes are tender. Drain and set aside to cool.

2. Add the mustard, sour cream and mayonnaise into a large bowl and stir to combine well. Afterwards, add the salt and pepper.

3. Stir in potatoes, celery, pickles, parsley and green onions to the mixture, stir while adding each item, taste and adjust seasoning by adding salt and pepper as required. Serve into plates, enjoy!


## Roasted Beet Salad
Yields: 8 servings

Preparation time: 10 minutes + 3 hours marinating time

Cooking time: 1 hour

**Ingredients:**

1 bunch of spinach, stems removed, sliced thinly

1½ pounds baby beets with greens attached

1 head garlic, halved

4 tablespoons extra-virgin olive oil, divided into 2

¾ teaspoon kosher salt, divided

1 cup distilled white vinegar

¼ cup sugar

½ cup toasted walnuts, chopped finely

¼ cup red onion, chopped finely

¼ cup fresh dill, chopped

**Instructions:**

1. Preheat oven to 325°F.

2. Rinse beets with tap water, cut off greens and separate the leaves from the stalk, set stalk and greens aside.

3. Next, place halved garlic, beets, ½ teaspoon of salt and 2 tablespoons of oil into a baking pan, cover with aluminum foil and place in the oven to roast for about 1 hour until tender. Remove from the oven and set aside to cool.

4. Transfer roasted beet to a flat surface and chop roughly, combine sugar and vinegar into a large bowl, whisk thoroughly.

5. Squeeze the garlic cloves into the bowl and add chopped beet. Cover in foil and marinate for about 3-4 hours at room temperature.

6. Place beet stalk on a flat surface and chop finely, slice the greens and transfer to a large bowl. After 3 hours, remove the beets from the pickling liquid and place in the bowl.

7. Drizzle about ¼ cup of pickling liquid over the bowl of beets. Next, add the red onion, dilli, walnuts, oil and salt and toss for about 30 seconds to combine. Serve divided into plates, enjoy!

# Curry-Berry Turkey Salad

Yields: 2 servings

Preparation time: 10 minutes

**Ingredients:**

2 tbsp of golden raisins

2 tsp of sugar

1/2 cup mayonnaise

3/4 tsp of curry powder

1/2 tsp of lime zest, grated

2 tsp of lime juice

1/4 tsp of salt

2 sliced celery ribs

1/4 cup red onion, chopped

2 cups of cubed turkey breast, cooked

3 cups fresh strawberries, sliced

**Instructions:**

1. Mix in the sugar, mayonnaise, curry, lime zest, lime juice and salt in a small bowl until well combined.

2. In a different larger bowl, combine the celery, onions, raisins and turkey. Pour the sugar and mayonnaise mixture over the turkey mixture and toss repeatedly to coat.

3. Add strawberries and serve, enjoy!

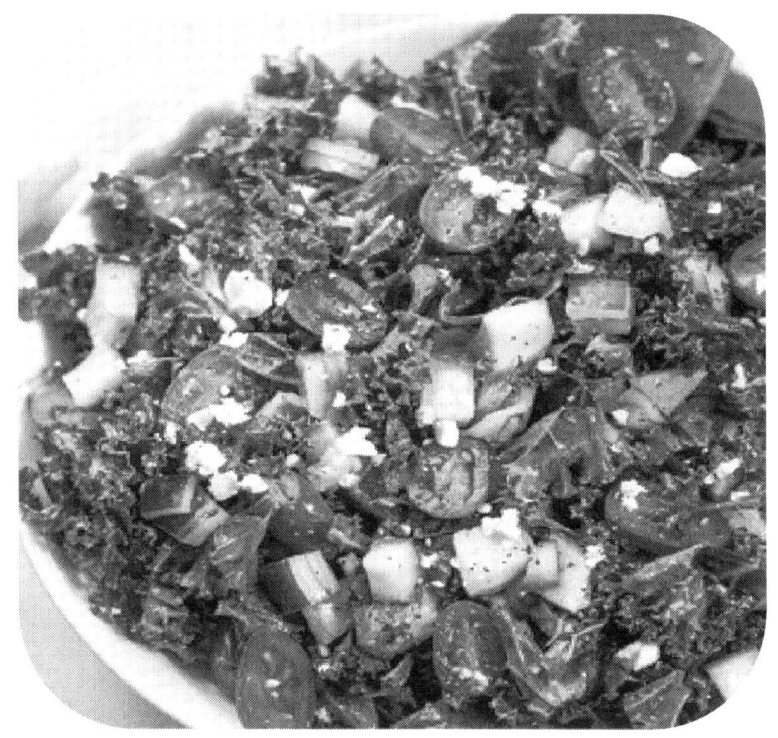

Greek Salad

## Healthiest Greek Salad

Yields: 3 servings

Preparation time: 10 minutes

**Ingredients:**

For the Dressing:

1/4 cup of olive oil

1/2 tsp of salt

2 tbsp of red wine vinegar

1/4 tsp of pepper

**For the Salad:**

4 cups of romaine lettuce

1 large cucumber

1/2 cup of kalamata olives

4 large sized tomatoes, sliced

1 large onion, sliced

4oz of feta cheese, diced

1 lemon, zested

1 tsp of dried oregano

**Instructions:**

1. For the dressing, mix the olive oil, vinegar, salt and pepper into a small bowl to combine well.

2. In a separate larger bowl, mix in all ingredients for the salad, combine with the dressing and toss repeatedly to coat well. Serve, enjoy!

# Kale Salad with Honey Lemon Dressing

Yields: 3 servings

Preparation time: 15 minutes

**Ingredients:**

For the Salad Dressing:

4 tablespoon of fresh lemon juice

2 tablespoon of extra virgin olive oil

1 tablespoon of honey

1/2 teaspoon of salt

1/8 teaspoon of black pepper

**Ingredients for Kale Salad:**

1 cup of pecans, shelled

8 cups loosely packed kale, chopped into 1/2 inch pieces

1 cup of dried cranberries

1 small red onion, sliced thinly

1 crisp apple

1 ripe and firm peas

**Instructions:**

1. Add all dressing ingredients into a bowl and stir vigorously, set aside.

2. Place pecans in a medium sized skillet over medium heat, heat for about 5 minutes until the pecans turn brown and fragrant, stir frequently. Remove from heat and set aside.

3. Combine the kale and cranberries into a large bowl, lightly drizzle with the dressing ingredients and stir repeatedly to coat well. Refrigerate for about 3 hours or more.

4. Add pecans, onions, apples and pears before serving, toss repeatedly to combine, enjoy!

# Healthiest Greek Salad

Yields: 3 servings

Preparation time: 10 minutes

**Ingredients:**

For the Dressing:

1/4 cup of olive oil

1/2 tsp of salt

2 tbsp of red wine vinegar

1/4 tsp of pepper

**For the Salad:**

4 cups of romaine lettuce

1 large cucumber

1/2 cup of kalamata olives

4 large sized tomatoes, sliced

1 large onion, sliced

4oz of feta cheese, diced

1 lemon, zested

1 tsp of dried oregano

**Instructions:**

1. For the dressing, mix the olive oil, vinegar, salt and pepper into a small bowl to combine well.

2. In a separate larger bowl, mix in all ingredients for the salad, combine with the dressing and toss repeatedly to coat well. Serve, enjoy!

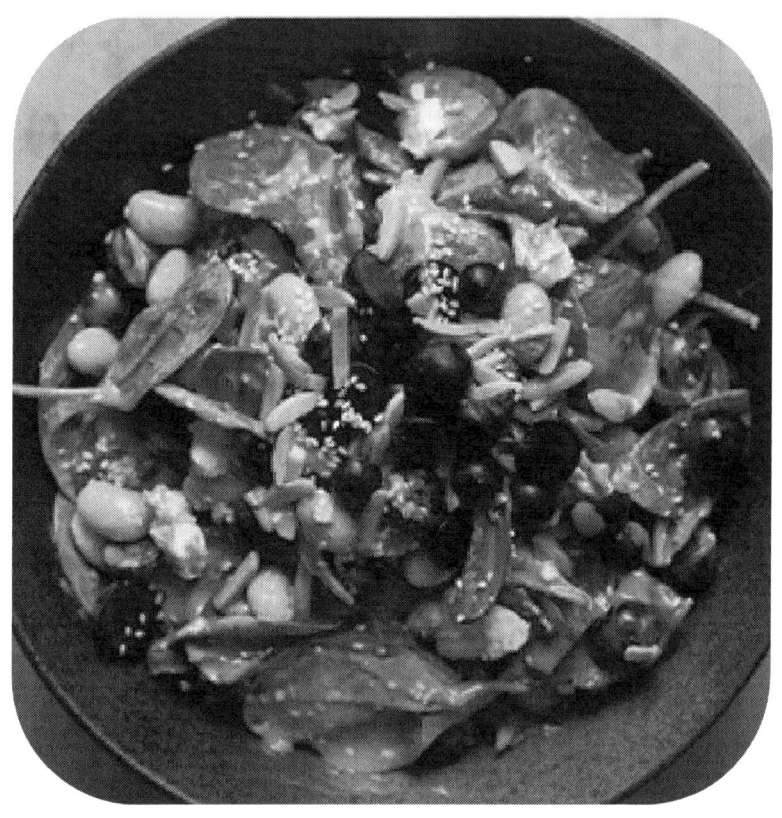

*Fig, Grape and Spinach Salad*

# Fig, Grape and Spinach Salad

Yields: 4 servings

Preparation time: 10 minutes

**Ingredients:**

3 figs, quartered

12 grapes, halved

1 cup of Spinach

1/4 cup walnuts

1/8 cup roasted pumpkin seeds

3 tbsp of balsamic vinegar

3 tbsp of extra virgin olive oil

1/4 tsp of salt

**Instructions:**

1. Mix the first 4 ingredients into a bowl.

2. In a smaller bowl, add the remaining ingredients and stir, combine dressing with the salad and toss repeatedly to coat well, serve.

# Smoothies, Shakes And Drinks

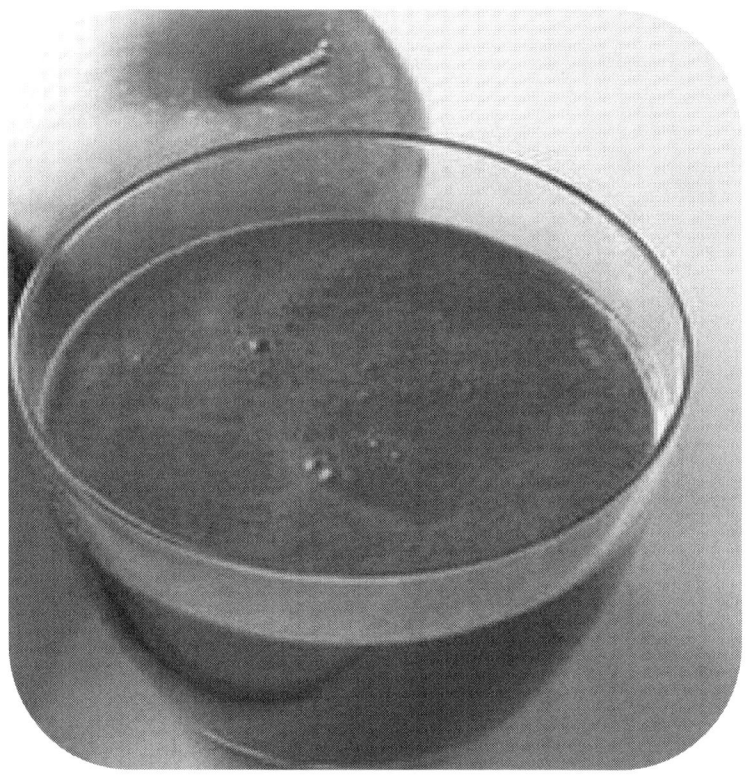

*Beet Carrot Apple Ginger Juice*

# Beet Carrot Apple Ginger Juice

Yields: 1 serving

Preparation time: 10 minutes

**Ingredients:**

4 medium sized-carrots, rinsed and scrubbed

2 handfuls of baby spinach

1 medium sized red beet

1 medium sized cucumber

1 lemon, rind removed

1 green apple, cored

1 piece of fresh ginger root

Pinch of sea salt

**Instructions:**

1. Push the ingredients through your juicer, and consume whole or strain with a fine mesh sieve.

# Almond Milk and Berry Smoothie

Preparation time: 10 minutes

Yield: 2 servings

**Ingredients:**

1/2 medium sized banana, diced into thick chunks

1/4 cup of blueberries, frozen

1/4 cup of strawberries, frozen

1/4 cup of mango, chopped

2 cups of chilled vanilla-flavored almond milk, unsweetened

**Instructions:**

1. Combine all ingredients into a blender and blend until well combined. Serve, enjoy!

# Cranberry pomegranate citrus mocktail

Yields: 4 servings

Preparation time: 10 minutes

**Ingredients:**

2 cups of ice, crushed

1 cup of pomegranate juice

½ cup of unsweetened cranberry juice

1/2 cup orange juice, squeezed freshly

1 cup of sparkling water

**Instructions:**

1. Combine all ingredients except the sparkling water into a pitcher and stir until well combined.

2. Divide the crushed ice into 4 glasses, add the sparkling water and pour in the mixture, stir. Enjoy!

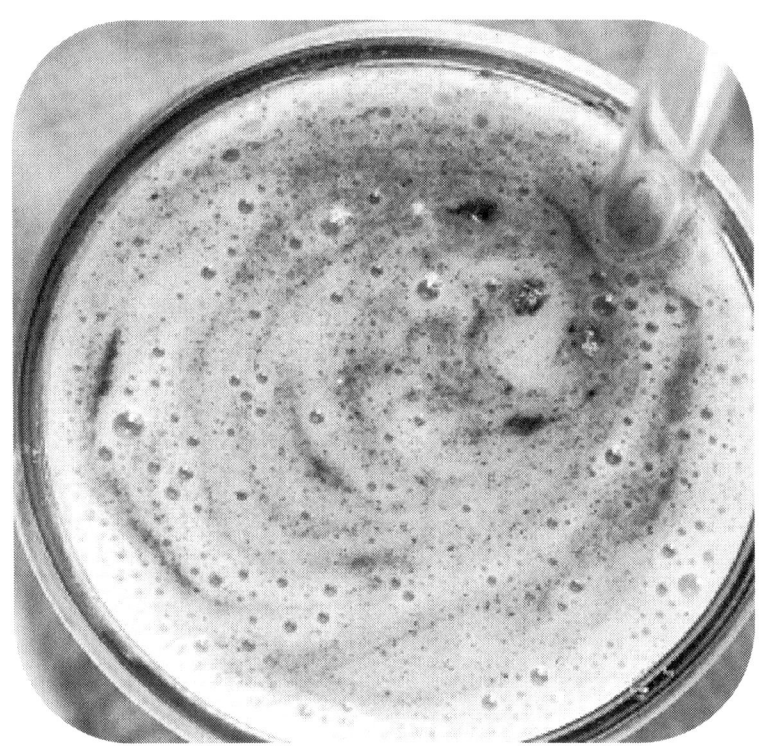

## Vanilla Cappuccino Protein Smoothie

Yields: 4 servings

Preparation time: 10 minutes

**Ingredients**

5.3 ounces of vanilla yogurt

2 shots of espresso

4 tablespoon of vanilla protein powder

2 cup of 2% fat milk

1/2 cup of ice.

**Instructions**

1. Combine all ingredients into a blender and blend until well combined. Serve, enjoy!

# Pumpkin Spice Latte Recipe

Yields: 4 servings

Preparation time: 10 minutes

**Ingredients:**

4 cups of almond milk

4 tablespoon of canned pumpkin puree

8 teaspoon of vanilla extract

2 teaspoon of pumpkin pie spice

1 cup of chilled espresso

4 teaspoon of honey

1/2 cup of ice cubes

Whipped cream

**Instructions:**

1. Add all ingredients apart from the ice cubes and whipped cream into a blender and blend until smooth, add ice cubes and blend some more.

2. Transfer contents into cups, top with whipped cream, enjoy!

# Healthy Shamrock Shake

Yields: 4 servings

Preparation time: 5 minutes

**Ingredients:**

4 cups of almond milk

1 avocado, pitted

4 handful of baby spinach

1 tsp of peppermint extract

20 soft Medjool date.

A handful of ice

**Instructions:**

1. Combine all ingredients into a blender and blend until smooth. Serve, enjoy!

# Creamy Banana Smoothie

Yields: 4 servings

Preparation time: 5 minutes

**Ingredients:**

4 large frozen banana

1/2 tsp of ground nutmeg

16 tbsp of walnuts

1.33 cup oats, quick oats

1 tsp of ground cinnamon

4 pinch of sea salt

1 tbsp of maple syrup

2 tsp of vanilla extract

3/4 cup  of almond milk

**Instructions:**

1. Combine all ingredients into a blender and blend until smooth. Serve, enjoy!

# Turmeric Tea

Yields: 2 servings

Preparation time: 5 minutes

**Ingredients:**

1 cup of water

1 cup of coconut milk

1 tbsp of ghee

1 tbsp of honey

1 tsp of turmeric powder

**Instructions:**

1. Combine the water and milk into a saucepan over low-medium heat and cook for 2 minutes, add the rest of the ingredients and cook for another 2 minutes. Stir frequently.

2. Pour into glasses. Enjoy!

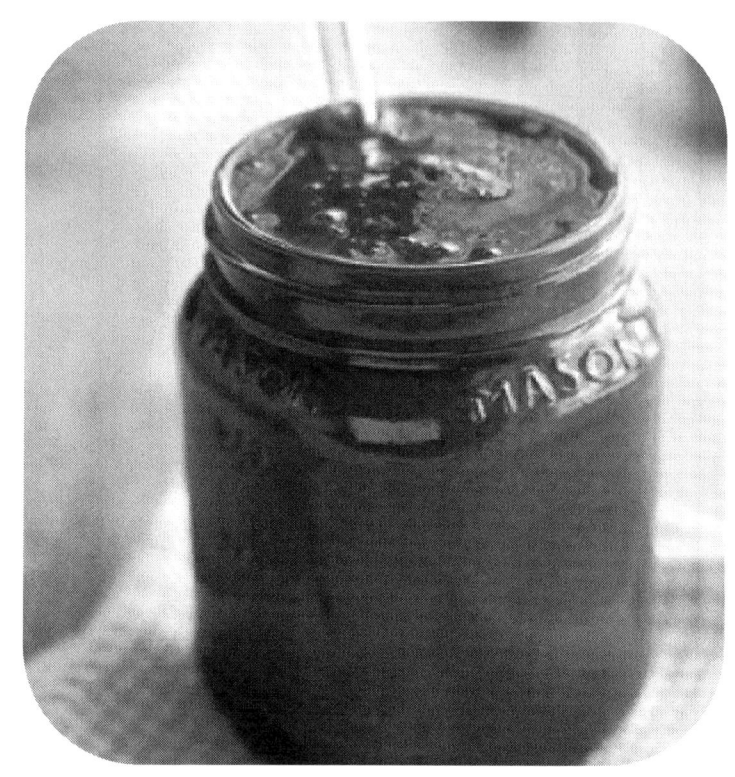

*Apple Berry Beet Smoothie*

# Apple Berry Beet Smoothie

Yields: 2 servings

Preparation time: 10 minutes

**Ingredients:**

1 1/2 cups of unsweetened coconut milk

1 small red beet, peeled and cut into wedges

1 1/2 cups of mixed berries, frozen

1 medium sized frozen apple, chopped into large pieces

1 tsp of vanilla extract

Walnuts to garnish

Honey optional

**Instructions:**

1. Combine all ingredients except the walnuts into a blender and blend until smooth. taste and a few teaspoons of honey if desired. Blend again for about 10 seconds and transfer to a jar and stand for a few minutes.

2. Serve garnished with walnuts, enjoy!

# Healthy Iced Coffee

Preparation time: 2 minutes

Yield: 1 serving

**Ingredients:**

1/2 cup of ice

1/2 cup of coffee, cold

1/2 cup of unsweetened almond milk

1 teaspoon of pure vanilla extract

**Instructions:**

1. First add ice then coffee, milk and vanilla extract into a glass

2. Stir to mix well, Enjoy!

# SNACKS

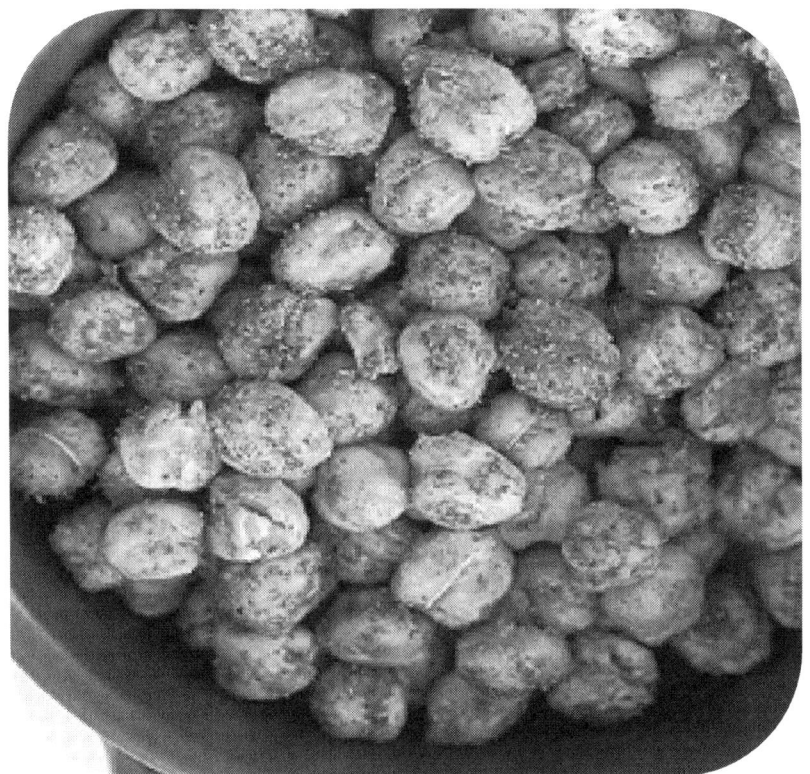

*Roasted chickpea*

# Apple Crumble

Yields: 6 servings

Preparation time:

Cooking time:

**Ingredients:**

For the filling;

6 medium apples, chopped

Generous splash of water

1 tsp of vanilla extract

1/2 tsp of ground cinnamon

**For the crumble topping;**

1 1/2 cups of rolled oats, organic

1/2 cup organic flaked coconut

1/2 tsp of ground cinnamon

1 tsp of vanilla extract paste

1-2 tbsp pure maple syrup (optional)

3-4 tbsp of coconut oil

**Instructions:**

1. Combine the apple, water, vanilla and cinnamon into a medium sized saucepan and cook for 20 minutes until the apples are soft and collapsed. Taste and adjust cinnamon as desired.

2. Place mixture into a baking dish, set aside.

**For the crumble:**

1. First, preheat oven to 320 F

2. Add all ingredients into a bowl, stir with your fingers to combine, then drizzle crumbs over the apple mixture.

3. Place in the oven and bake for 35 minutes until the crumble turns golden.

4. Transfer to a bowl and serve with Greek styled yoghurt. Enjoy!

## Roasted chickpea

Yields: 6 serving

Preparation time: 10 minutes

Cooking time: 30 minutes

**Ingredients:**

2 can of chickpeas, drained and rinsed

1 tbsp of olive oil

1 tsp of cumin

A sprinkle of garlic powder

A sprinkle of cayenne pepper

A sprinkle of sea salt

**Instructions:**

1. Preheat oven to 400 degrees.

2. Dry rinsed chickpeas by covering with paper towels, transfer to a bowl and add the remaining ingredients, stir to combine.

3. Transfer chickpeas to a baking sheet and bake for about 30 minutes, shake the baking sheet at 10 minutes intervals. Monitor to prevent excessive browning. Enjoy!

# Garlic Kale Chips

Yields: 4 serving

Preparation time: 10 minutes

Cooking time: 25 minutes

**Ingredients:**

1 bunch of curly kale, rinsed and dried, stalks removed, leaves chopped finely.

2 tbsp of olive oil

1 tsp of kosher salt

1/2 tsp of garlic powder

**Instructions:**

1. Preheat oven to 325F.

2. Combine chopped kale leaves and olive oil into a bowl; mix with your fingers to coat well.

3. Place kale leaves over two baking sheets, lightly drizzle salt and garlic powder then bake for 20 minutes, flip using a spatula after 10 minutes to ensure even baking. Bake until crisp, enjoy!

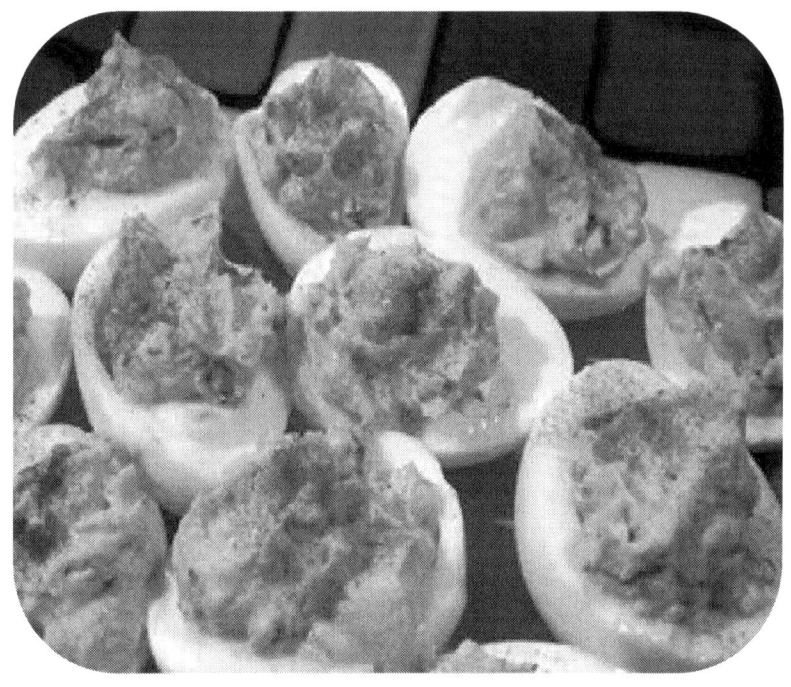

*Avocado Deviled Eggs*

## Avocado Deviled Eggs

Yields: 12 servings

Preparation time: 10 minutes

**Ingredients:**

6 hard-boiled eggs, peeled and halved

1 avocado peeled, pitted and diced

2 tsp of lime juice

3 slices of cooked turkey bacon, chopped and divided

2 1/2 tbsp of mayonnaise

1/8 tsp of cayenne pepper

1 clove of garlic, crushed

Salt

1 jalapeno pepper, sliced (optional)

**Instructions:**

1. Combine egg yolk, avocado, lime juice, 2/3 of turkey bacon, ,pepper ,garlic and salt into a bowl, stir until well combined.

2. Spoon filling into egg white, layer with reserved turkey bacon and jalapeno pepper, enjoy!


## Blueberry Coconut Granola Bars
Yields: 15 bars

Preparation time: 10 minutes

Cooking time: 40 minutes

**Ingredients:**

1/2 cup of toasted coconut, shredded

3-1/2 cups whole grain oats

1/4 cup of whole wheat flour

1/2 cup of puffed rice cereal

1 cup of dried blueberries

1/3 cup of brown sugar

1/2 tsp of kosher salt

1/2 cup of coconut oil, melted

1/2 cup of honey

1 1/2 tsp of coconut extract

1/2 tsp of vanilla extract

1/4 slivered almonds optional

**Instructions:**

1. Preheat oven to 325F

2. Coat a large sized baking sheet with cooking spray, line with parchment paper and set aside.

3. Next stir in the oats, cereal, wheat, coconut, sugar, salt and blueberries into a large bowl. In a different bowl, add the remaining ingredients and stir. Combine both ingredients into the larger bowl and stir to mix well.

4. Place the mixture into the baking sheet, transfer to the oven and bake for about 30 minutes or until bars turn golden brown. Remove from the oven and cool

5. Cut into bars once cooled, enjoy!

Orange Salsa

Yields: 6 servings

Preparation time: 10 minutes + 1 hour chill time

**Ingredients:**

2 large oranges, peeled and cut into chunks

1 tomato, seeded and diced

1/2 cup of red onion, minced

1 tbsp of apple juice

1 tsp of orange zest, grated

1 tsp of garlic, minced

1/4 jalapeno pepper, chopped finely

1/2 tsp of fresh ginger root, chopped finely

1 pinch salt

1 tbsp of fresh cilantro, chopped finely

**Instructions:**

1. Combine all ingredients into a bowl, refrigerate for about 1 hour until chilled, Add cilantro and stir before serving. Enjoy!

Easy Guacamole
Yields: 16 servings

Preparation time:

Cooking time:

**Ingredients:**

2 avocados, peeled and mashed

1 small onion, chopped finely

1 clove of garlic, minced

1 ripe  medium sized tomato, chopped

1 lime, juiced

Salt and pepper to taste

**Instructions:**

1. Combine all ingredients into a bowl, refrigerate for about 1 hour until chill. Enjoy!

The End

Printed in Great Britain
by Amazon